WALKING

WALKING

JOHN PLEAS, Ph.D.

W·W·NORTON & COMPANY   New York · London

Published simultaneously in Canada by Penguin Books Canada Ltd.,
2801 John Street, Markham, Ontario L3R 1B4.
Printed in the United States of America.

The text of this book is composed in Compano, with
display type set in Eras. Composition and
manufacturing by the Haddon Craftsmen, Inc.
Book design by Jacques Chazaud

Library of Congress Cataloging-in-Publication Data

Pleas, John.
Walking.

1. Walking.   2. Physical fitness.   3. Reducing
exercises.   I. Title.
RA781.65.P57   1987   613.7'1   86–23668

ISBN 0-393-02446-6

W. W. Norton & Company, Inc.
500 Fifth Avenue, New York, N. Y. 10110
W. W. Norton & Company Ltd.
37 Great Russell Street, London WC1B 3 NU

1 2 3 4 5 6 7 8 9 0

Contents

Foreword

John Pleas is more than a friend and colleague. For me, as well as for thousand of others, he is an inspiration.

When John walks into a room, the atmosphere suddenly seems lighter, filled with good spirits and energy. If you are fortunate enough to hear him lecture on physical fitness, or to see or hear him in one of his radio or TV interviews, I assure you that your feet will start to tingle and twitch. You will not be able to restrain yourself. Soon you will be itching to get up out of your chair and walk somewhere, just to experience the footing he describes.

While John was the co-director of the Vanderbilt Weight Management Program (1977–1984), he not only introduced me and hundreds of our weight management group participants to the benefits of walking for weight management, but he became the Pied Piper of Nashville. On his 24-hour birthday walk, which he briefly mentions in the book, hundreds of Nashvillians joined him, as I did, for a part of the journey. It was a memorable day for all of us as John traveled 'round the clock, covering his favorite routes and visiting some of his favorite haunts where he occasionally stopped for a cup of coffee and chatted with a few of his many friends.

Of course you can expect to find the best technical advice about walking in *Walking*. And walking is, in my opinion, the safest and most convenient activity for weight control, cardiovascular health, and all-around physical well-being. If you have forty or fifty pounds to lose, the key to keeping that weight off once lost is with a 45-minute walk each day.

But *Walking* is about much more than walking. In the first edition of his book, John wrote an inscription to me: "This book is not really about walking. It is about growth, success, determination, and dedication. It's about an 'I can' and an 'I will' attitude, and moving to the beat of your own drum. Walking is simply a convenient vehicle." John is a living expression of all of these attitudes in his own life, and walking certainly is his personal vehicle.

If you have been saying things such as "I can't seem to get motivated when it comes to exercise," or "I'm trying to get active, but something always seems to come up to interfere with my best intentions," read *Walking*. John's spirit is infectious. You will catch the bug. As you follow his advice, I think you, too, will find how joyful it is to be a vigorous and healthy human animal. You may also find, as John intends, that walking will be an experience in the growth and development of positive self-regard. Together, the physical and psychological benefits of walking will inspire you and sustain your motivation.

Walking is a book for everyone, but I want to recommend it especially to my professional colleagues in every area of health promotion in which exercise and weight management play a role. The book contains some simple to implement self-tests of fitness and then outlines several walking programs, each at a different level of intensity and duration for persons at different levels of fitness. There are programs suitable for beginners as well as persons at higher levels of fitness. Thus the book will be an excellent companion, supplementing your efforts to encourage your program participants in their pursuit of a healthier, happier, more active life-style.

And now, read on. As John says, you are about to discover that walking can be a "moving experience"!

Martin Katahn, Ph.D.
author of *The Rotation Diet* and
Director of the Vanderbilt University
Weight Management Program

Acknowledgments

I want to thank Dr. Robert Orlando, Ms. Katherine Smits, and Ms. Dona Tapp for sharing their ideas with me on the central focus of this book. Dona also served as my editor and I am very grateful to her for the exceptional guidance and technical assistance she provided.

Special appreciation is also given to the hundreds of walkers over the years who shared their walking stories with me and to my colleagues, Dr. Martin Katahn and Dr. Kenneth Wallston, who made helpful suggestions on the manuscript.

Thanks to Chandra, my daughter, for her patience on those occasions when my work on the book took up portions of our valuable time together.

Finally, I am deeply indebted to my loving wife, Katherine, who urged me to persist when I became discouraged by reminding me that walking, writing, and other goals in life are attainable when taken One Step At A Time.

WALKING

1

Introduction

Americans are in the midst of a fitness revolution. Books on exercise and physical fitness now rival those on sex as the No. 1 best sellers. Our national preoccupation with exercise is also reflected in our purchase of exercise equipment, our memberships in health spas, and our increasing pursuit of leisure activities.

According to Hofstra University sociologist Natalie Allon, Americans spent $100 million on the purchase of exercise equipment in 1976 and $220 million on memberships in health spas and reducing salons in the same year. A recent report by *U.S. News and World Report* indicates that leisure spending (hiking, camping, movies, and other recreational activities) increased from $58.3 billion in 1964 to $180 billion in 1978. In the past few years, the trend has continued at a rate that goes even beyond what most sociologists, economists, exercise physiologists, and fitness buffs might have predicted.

Despite this emphasis on exercise and fitness, and the increased purchase of jogging suits and shoes, exercise and physical fitness are still part of an elusive dream—an exercise (or non-exercise, actually) in futility. Finding an exercise that requires minimal time and effort and yet yields a high payoff and a guarantee of a body that is fit and beautiful continues to elude most Americans.

Continuing on the present course will result in the same

consequences tomorrow as we are experiencing today: a high drop-out rate from formal exercise programs, a waste of our money, increased medical and physical complications due to injury (mostly because of our propensity for instant success), and, ultimately, a negative attitude toward exercise. Our present approach to exercise and fitness must be tempered by a more commonsense approach to avoid these pitfalls. *Walking,* a book about experiencing the joy of walking and changing your sedentary life-style, has been written as an alternative to the current exercise hodgepodge sweeping the country.

Walking is written from a personal and professional perspective. It is personal in the sense that I am a passionate walker. I average 12 miles a day Monday through Friday, 22 miles on Saturday, and I relax on Sunday by walking 15. To me, walking is as good for the mind as for the body. Walking is an integral part of my life. Last year I celebrated my 42nd birthday by going for a 24-hour walk. That walk, which covered 79 miles, was a part of what has now become an annual event in Nashville: The John Pleas Birthday Walkathon. Each year, more and more people in the community join my celebration of life. No ice cream! No cake! No contributions for presents! Just a sharing of the joy!

The professional perspective is from having read hundreds of articles and books on walking and physical fitness for the past four years and from being co-director of a weight management program at a major university during this period. As a weight management group leader, I have prescribed walking as the core physical fitness activity for hundreds of moderately and massively obese clients. I am the walking leader for two groups that walk at different times in different sections of Nashville every Saturday morning. In addition, I have developed successful walking programs for a number of weight management groups in other communities. Dedicated walkers from these groups report that walking has enhanced their lives.

I have written this book with three purposes in mind: to

share my personal and professional views on walking with a wider audience than the Nashville community; to provide basic self-help information to get each of you started; and to inspire you to experience personally the beneficial effects of walking—which, ultimately, is the key to your continuing to walk after the novelty has worn off.

Walking begins with a brief history of walking and its popularity and tells you why walking is for everyone. Questions asked frequently by new walkers and skeptics are answered, and there are tips on the when, where, and why of walking, on wearing apparel, and on walking aids. I go on to discuss some of the factors associated with getting the most out of each step and the physical, psychological, and financial benefits that can be gained through walking. Finally, recommendations are presented to alleviate common physical complaints that may occur, as well as motivational tips to maintain your interest in walking as a lifelong physical activity. While the major focus of the book is on experiencing what walking is, a gradual and progressive walking program is included in the appendix for those of you who are interested in achieving a high level of fitness from walking.

I would be remiss if I did not address your expectations that walking might change your life completely or solve the major world problems. Let me state at the beginning, then, what you cannot expect as a result of following my suggestions that you walk more. You cannot expect:

- a Hollywood contract within the first year
- a 10-pound weight loss in a single week
- total immunity from disease
- reconciliation of irreconcilable differences
- eternal life
- an appearance on "The Tonight Show"
- first place in the next Miss America or Mr. Universe contest
- straight As without studying

- that people will like you better
- 1st place in the 1980 Olympic fast-walking event
- a 50% increase in annual salary (of course, this might come later, as you gain more energy and confidence)

If you have any of these expectations for instant success, this book is not for you.

Since walking is active rather than passive, you must participate to receive optimal benefits. So if you are ready for a different approach and a rewarding experience that may change some important aspects of your life—irrespective of your age, sex, race, occupation, education, or income level—then this book is for you. Your expectations will be met if you are interested in becoming involved in a free, individually tailored, noncompetitive, lifelong, safe physical activity that has worked for millions through the years.

Walk with me through the pages of this book, read and do, and experience for yourself what walking is. A word of caution though:

WALKING IS A MOVING EXPERIENCE
THAT CAN LEAD TO A POSITIVE ADDICTION

2

The Silent Majority

The unearthing of the pelvic bones of the early hominid *Australopithecus,* with an upright posture and bipedal gait, suggests that the ability to walk on two legs occurred approximately 4 million years ago. It has been a source of interest ever since. The first group to study walking was the Greeks. These scholars were interested in understanding the structural and functional aspects of the human body in motion. In fact, the Greek philosopher Aristotle spent countless hours observing the movement of the human body and became known as the "Father of Kinesiology." His study of the movement of the body was congruent with the prevalent philosophy in Greece during the period that emphasized the development of the total person. With the decline of the Greek culture and the ushering in of the Early Christian Age and the Middle Ages, the development of the body and the pursuit of leisure were de-emphasized.

Man's awakening to the pleasures and benefits of walking was revived during the Renaissance period, and it continued unabated into the nineteenth and twentieth centuries. The pleasure derived from walking is evident in eighteenth- and nineteenth-century literature, which was characterized by the poems and essays of such noted authors as Thoreau, Carlyle, Wordsworth, and Taylor. Words such as path, road, highway, street, foot, and trod were quite prevalent. An excerpt from "The Open Road" by Walt Whitman is characteristic of some of the poems during this period:

Afoot and light-hearted I take to the open road,
Healthy, free, the world before me,
The long brown path before me leading wherever I choose.
Henceforth I ask not good-fortune, I myself am good-fortune,
Henceforth I whimper no more, postpone no more, need nothing,
Done with indoor complaints, libraries, querulous criticisms,
Strong and content I travel the open road.

Writings in the first half of the twentieth century reflect America's preoccupation with wars, depression, and the basic issues of survival. Gasoline rationing necessitated that man walk more during this time. Newspaper articles on the joy of walking, and editorials encouraging Americans to walk more, were commonplace. With the advent of automobiles, airplanes, buses, and trains after World War II, and an increase in the gross national product, walking as a popular mode of transportation was abandoned by many. There were still a number of Americans, though, who refused the new modes of transportation and who, even though they had access to automobiles, continued to walk for sheer pleasure.

Even today, in spite of our advanced technology, a number of Americans are continuing to walk, and the trend is growing. Several years ago, a survey of leisure activities revealed that those activities related to walking were the most popular, with 96.7 million people walking or jogging, 61.9 million going nature walking, and 28.1 million hiking and backpacking. More recently, walking was substantiated as the most popular physical activity in America. The 1979 Perrier Study on Fitness in America, which included a survey by Lou Harris, revealed that, despite the boom in jogging, walking is still the most popular and preferred physical activity in America.

Not Just for the Healthy

There are 34 million walkers in America, as compared with 17 million joggers; thus walkers are in the majority. Are you surprised? Probably. Because walkers tend to do their own thing fairly quietly. Who are these people who comprise this silent majority? They are young, old, rich, poor, black, white, healthy, recuperating from illness or surgery; they live in the country and in cities; they walk by day and they walk by night. As the composition of this silent majority suggests, walking is for everyone.

Hippocrates, the Father of Medicine, recommended daily walks for one of his patients in the fourth century B.C., and still today, walking is one of the major exercise prescriptions recommended by physicians for patients suffering from arthritis, diabetes, cardiovascular and circulatory problems, obesity, ulcers, migraine headaches, and a host of other medical problems. In addition, walking is the exercise of choice during pregnancy and is even helpful during labor. In a recent study conducted in England, expectant women who walked during labor had fewer complications during delivery than did non-walkers and their newborn babies were found to be less likely to exhibit abnormalities in the fetal heartbeat.

There has also been a progressive tendency in recent years to get people back on their feet quickly following childbirth and surgery. Thirty years ago, women were encouraged to stay in bed several days after giving birth; surgery patients were similarly urged to stay in bed and rest quietly in order to build up their strength. Today, the postoperative plan is usually straightforward: Get the patients moving, get them active, get them on their feet! Prolonged bed rest has physical, psychological, and financial ramifications that in most cases are contrary to the ultimate goal of medical treatment —a return to an active life-style.

From the physical perspective, muscle tone and bulk diminish with disuse and the blood has to work against gravitational forces while a patient is bedridden. A number of exercises are recommended during recuperation that are helpful in preventing degenerative changes: gentle massage to improve peripheral circulation, deep breathing exercises, postural exercises, and range-of-motion exercises to increase the flexibility of joints. In addition, walking, which engages the long muscles of the leg, improves circulation and prevents the pooling of blood in the lower extremities. With the increased circulation of the blood, oxygen is utilized more efficiently by the body, and, more important, vital nutrients are transported throughout the body to hasten recovery.

The psychological and financial benefits of walking as soon as possible after surgery or while recuperating are also worth mentioning. Early mobility increases a patient's sense of general well-being, self-confidence, and independence. In addition, when patients are able to do more for themselves, boredom and anxiety are reduced, fear of exertion is removed, and morale is improved. With respect to the financial benefits associated with getting up and around early, studies have shown that care for bedridden patients costs more than care for ambulatory patients. In addition, the longer a patient is bedridden, the longer and slower the recovery time, and thus the higher the overall cost of hospitalization. Of course you will not always have a choice about how early you can get out of bed, but when you do, EXERCISE IT!

If you or a friend or family member are recuperating from surgery right now, a physical therapist should be by your bedside in a few days. If not, assert yourself and ask your doctor for some light exercises to speed your recovery. And if you're not already walking, ask your doctor when you can!

Walking through the Ages

The proportion of the American population over the age of 65 is growing rapidly. In 1900, there were 3 million Americans 65 or older; in 1975, the aged population exceeded 23 million; and by 1990, the number is expected to reach 30 million. What is the physical activity prognosis for this increasing population of older, somewhat sedentary persons? And what is the recommended physical activity for this population? At a recent three-day conference sponsored by the National Institutes of Health and entitled "Exercise in Aging—Its Role in Prevention of Physical Decline," researchers agreed that:

> Walking is the most effective form of exercise . . . and the only one that you can safely follow all the years of your life.

(Somehow I expect you were not surprised at their recommendation.)

Quite simply, walking is a safe, simple, and easy exercise for the elderly whereby they can receive the psychological benefits (better self-image, increased zest for life, increased vigor) and the physical benefits (cardiovascular fitness, improved muscle tone, greater endurance, increased metabolic rate, increased work capacity). Yet an examination of the life-style of most Americans, and the elderly in particular, reveals that walking decreases with age. This does not have to be the case.

A brief look into the lives of Jesse Hyde and Adomar Varnar highlights the importance of walking as a lifelong activity for the elderly. Hyde, a retired insurance man, made the headlines several years ago when he celebrated his 75th birthday with a 24-hour hike of 75 miles. Varnar, a Lithuanian immigrant who celebrated his 100th birthday recently, attributed his longevity to the following factors: moderation in life-style, plenty of interest, a balanced diet that includes non-canned food without artificial preservatives, plenty of fresh fruit juices, and, last but not least, WALKING.

Then there is the report of Ed Coleman, from a rural county near Spartansburg, South Carolina. Ed walked 2 ½ miles to cast his vote in a recent election. It took him 2 hours, but he was determined to participate in the political progress of his nation. Ed Coleman is 103 years old.

What about elderly women? Sarah Dale Mannakee and Rose Freeman are both 103, and their secret for a long and healthy life is similar: staying busy and interested in a variety of projects, doing missionary work and helping others, and . . . WALKING. You do not have to wait until you are 100 years old to enjoy walking. Ask Rose Kennedy or Greta Garbo.

Special Benefits for Women

For men and women alike, then, walking is related to maintaining a long and healthy life. But for women, there are additional physical benefits that can be achieved in the advancing years.

The human skeleton achieves its greatest mass at about age 25, and as a weight-bearing organ, it maintains maximum efficiency for the next 20 to 25 years. After the age of 45, small changes occur in the joints and spine. From age 50 on, it is normal for a woman to lose approximately .5% of the total skeletal mass per year (bone loss in men is usually less than .5% and often does not begin until age 65 to 70). Consequently, all elderly persons, but particularly women, become increasingly susceptible to serious fractures as a result of a slight fall. In fact, fracture of the hip is one of the few age-related diseases that is more frequent among women than among men. Walking can decrease the probability of fractures by improving agility and balance. Recovery is also hastened by the increase in resiliency as a result of walking.

Another problem involving the skeletal system that is peculiar to women is osteoporisis. Osteoporosis, which primarily affects white females over the age of 50, is a bone disease that results in a bone loss of 1% a year instead of .5% a year as mentioned above. Moreover, there is mounting evidence from medical researchers that extreme muscular inactivity results in demineralization of bone tissue, and lack of exercise appears to play a role in the rapidity with which osteoporosis develops. Bone, like other parts of the body, is made up of living tissue that regenerates its own cells as they die and retains the capacity to repair itself, even into old age. Thus the constant rubbing of the long muscles against the bone, which occurs while walking, aids in the production of bone cells and makes bones less brittle. Walking is one of the exercises frequently recommended for the treatment and prevention of osteoporosis.

The conclusion is clear. Elderly persons can receive tremendous physical benefits and become less susceptible to injuries by walking more. A few basic questions here: Do you want to walk more? What are some of the reasons you are giving yourself for not walking more? Unsafe streets? A fear of walking alone? Where there's a will, there's a way.

People Need People

Walking clubs exist for the elderly in many cities and, in growing numbers, senior citizen organizations are enlisting community organizations and youth from the community to provide such services for the elderly. Recently, a sorority at the University of Alabama in Tuscaloosa joined hands with Project Focus in a service project involving the elderly. Each of nine sororities in a Pan Hellenic Council was assigned an elderly person to call on and walk with at least once a week and was expected to call on its adopted client to socialize during inclement weather. Is there a college in your area? Is there some other group of people who would be interested in providing this kind of support? Is it possible to form a walking group specifically for the elderly in your community? Could you organize it?

Can you get a family member to stop by your house or apartment three times a week for 30 minutes to go for a walk with you? Have you asked? Assert yourself and see what happens. If all else fails, advertise in the newspaper and see if you can get someone to come by and walk with you.

What? Oh, I'm sorry. I've been so busy talking to the 65 and over group that I've ignored you. Just stick with me another paragraph or so, because I have an assignment for all of you.

When you enlist the company of others you will find that the people you get to walk with you will probably get as much out of going for the walk as you. Tell your friends and family that, as much as you enjoy their coming to visit, you would enjoy it even more if they would come prepared to walk while they visit. Thus you may discover what Varnar, the 75-mile birthday walker, and Joseph Hyde, the 103-year-old voter, and the two praying and walking church women have known all along . . . that walking is a practical, purposeful, and pleasant physical activity that endures through the ages.

The list of persons who have joined the silent majority is endless. Look out your window in the morning. Go to the parks in the late evening. Observe people during the lunch hour. You will see the silent majority—not in jogging suits, but walking gracefully down the street. But why wait for tomorrow and observe others? Today is your day to join the silent majority. The walk you are about to take can make a difference in your life. It is the first test to see if you are willing to give yourself a chance to experience the joys of walking.

Assignment: Take a Walk

As soon as you finish this section, I want you to put the book down and go for a 5- to 10-minute stroll. Take the kettle off the stove, turn off all electrical appliances, get up and go out the door. But first, leave a message for your wife, husband, children, friends, or boss. Just say GONE WALKING. Walk around the block. Walk around the yard. If you cannot leave the house, walk in and around all the rooms, stairs, and hallways throughout the house three times without stopping. If you are an invalid or convalescent, stretch and wiggle your toes, tense your thigh and calf muscles, close your eyes, and go for an imaginary walk.

Do	**Don't**
Leave a message	Overdress—less is best
Walk at a moderate pace	Walk too far
Wear your most comfortable shoes	Stop and talk
Focus on enjoyment, not speed	Put it off until tomorrow

READY? Good. When you get back, elevate your feet while you complete the questionnaire on the next page.

Hey! Don't turn that page yet. I said AFTER you walk! If you're going to cheat, there is something I think you should consider: You'll be cheating yourself more than you'll be cheating me. I already KNOW about the joys of walking!

Assessment of Your Leisurely Stroll

Did you enjoy your brief walk?	yes	no
Were there other people walking?	yes	no
Were the people you saw congenial?	yes	no
Did you notice anything different in your environment while you were walking?	yes	no
Was your walk refreshing and did you feel more relaxed afterwards?	yes	no
Did you find that walking temporarily distracted you from a problem that had been on your mind?	yes	no
Did you find that walking helped you solve a problem?	yes	no
Were you able to cope better with some situation after completing your walk?	yes	no
Did you notice that you had more energy to complete some task upon returning?	yes	no
Was your mental attitude better when you completed your walk?	yes	no
If you went for a walk alone, did you enjoy the solitude and serenity?	yes	no
Were you able to accomplish a specific task during your walk? For instance, picking up items from the store? Getting the mail? Saying hello to a neighbor you hadn't seen for months?	yes	no

The purpose of this simple questionnaire was to acquaint you with just a few of the benefits that can be received from a brief walk. Count the number of times you checked yes. If you checked yes only once, your brief walk was beneficial. As you continue going for a walk, your personal list of benefits will increase. If you have doubts about this assertion, go for a 15- to 20-minute walk every day for the next month and then answer the questionnaire again. In the meantime, let me answer a few of the questions that new walkers and skeptics frequently ask.

3

Common Questions

Question: Is it true that I have to walk 35 miles to lose a pound?

Answer: Theoretically, this is true. One pound is equal to 3500 calories, and 1 mile of walking at a brisk pace will burn up approximately 100 calories. If you multiply 35 miles times 100 calories, the total will be 3500 calories, or 1 pound. However, this multiplication procedure is a very simplistic approach and does not take into consideration several fundamental factors: For one, you would not attempt to walk that many miles at one time, but would work toward a cumulative goal over a period of time. Second, the speed at which you walk is a factor. Walking speed is related to your heart rate, your heart rate is related to your metabolism, and your metabolism is related to the burning of fat. Thus walking faster will elevate your heart rate and basal metabolism and will help you burn fat more efficiently. Third, the thermogenetic effect as a result of walking has a carryover effect after you complete your walk. Consequently, 12 to 24 hours after you finish walking, your metabolism stays elevated and you are still burning up more calories while sitting than you would have if you had not gone for a walk. Finally, in most cases, you would not try to lose weight just by walking, with no other changes in your routine. Although it is possible to do that over a long period of time, the recommended weight loss procedure is to engage in a combined approach of gradually reducing your caloric intake and increasing your energy expenditure.

A 20-minute walk each day with your caloric intake held constant will result in a 10-pound weight loss in a year, which is a sensible approach to weight loss. However, if you want to lose a substantial amount of weight in a short time, you will have to cut calories as well.

Q: Will walking and other physical activities make me hungry?

A: Walking and other forms of continuous activity will not make you hungry. If you are hungry after completing a brisk 15- to 20-minute walk, you were probably hungry before you started walking. In all likelihood, eating after walking or after participating in some other kind of physical activity is just a bad habit that you have developed over the years. Ask any athlete if he/she is hungry after competing in a sporting event. Thirsty? Yes! Hungry? No! Brisk walking acts on the body to reduce hunger; it does not increase hunger.

Q: I am a female and am concerned that walking and jogging will turn me into a jock. Will walking make me have bulging muscles?

A: Walking will not cause bulging muscles, nor will it turn you into a jock. (Come to think of it, I am not sure just what is so offensive about women jocks!) Walking will tone up your muscles, though, and fat tissue will be replaced with muscle tissue. The female hormonal system is different from that of males and has a built-in mechanism that prevents bulging muscles. Some women are predisposed, based on their body type, to have well-developed muscles in the calf, thigh, upper arm, and other regions, but most women do not have this body type. Your own body type (endomorph, mesomorph, ectomorph) has been determined genetically and hereditarily, and walking will only improve on what is already there.

Q: I have heard that walking will only help a person lose weight from the waist down, and most of my excess weight is concentrated in the abdominal region. Shouldn't I do spot exercises instead of walking?

A: The muscle metabolism that occurs with the elevation of the heart rate benefits the total body, and you will begin losing weight where most of the fat deposits are laid down. Thus, the weight loss benefits from walking are not just from the waist down. I have treated obese clients who lost inches by walking even though they did not lose pounds. I have also seen people lose 50 to 60 pounds and have to purchase shoes one or two sizes smaller. This redistribution of weight and substantial weight loss in a particular area was not the result of spot exercising.

In an extreme case, one participant in my weight management program told me that he had lost 60 pounds several years ago and had to have his dentures replaced. Finally, as one physical fitness authority has pointed out, if spot exercises worked, people who chew gum would have slim jaws. A quick tally of the gum chewers you know will probably reveal that this is not the case.

Q: Why should I walk when I only want to lose 20 pounds?

A: There is no reason for you to walk if you want to lose 20 pounds—or any number of pounds. Caloric reduction will result in a weight loss; in fact, fasting will result in a very quick weight loss. Therefore, if you are only interested in losing weight, eat X number of calories, and in X number of days you will lose 20 pounds. However, if you are interested in the cosmetic effect of weight loss, in feeling your best, and in long-term weight loss and maintenance, then walking and other exercises will tone your muscles, reduce flabbiness in areas where excess adipose tissue has accumulated, and lead to permanent weight control.

Q: Isn't jogging better than walking?

A: According to Dr. Kenneth Cooper, author of *The New Aerobics,* some of the best exercises for achieving cardiovascular benefits are cross-country skiing, jogging, rowing, swimming, and, of course, walking. However, "better than" is relative. The best physical activity is (a) one that you can perform consistently, (b) one that will provide cardiovascular benefits, (c) one that can be easily incorporated into your present life-style, (d) one that can last a lifetime, and (e) one that you enjoy. If jogging meets these criteria, then jogging is better, but for many sedentary Americans, jogging is apparently not the answer. If you have access to a year-round swimming pool or warm beach, or can afford membership in a swimming club, swimming a certain number of laps four to five times a week at a certain speed is great. Cross-country skiing is even better, if your area of the country is one in which you can do it on a regular basis. Another option is to do a combination of all of the above. But whatever you choose, remember that enjoyment, consistency, and an elevated heart rate are the critical factors in a physically active life-style.

Q: My family was always inactive and I spent most of my childhood indoors practicing the piano, reading, and studying. Is it possible for me to become active with such an inactive history?

A: A body at rest tends to stay at rest unless some force acts upon it. This is an old physics principle and is another way of saying that inactivity breeds inactivity. You can overcome your sedentary life-style and become physically active. Furthermore, if you stick with an activity at an intense level long enough, you will become psychologically and physically addicted to the point where activity will breed activity. At this juncture the key for you is to adopt an *I Can and I Will* attitude. According to Dr. George Sheehan, a runner and a cardiologist, "the body is willing but it is the mind that is weak." Forget about the past and focus on the present and future and say *I Can and I Will.*

Q: Will walking make me tired and sleepy?

A: Although Charles Dickens used walking to cure his insomnia, walking as a general rule is an "upper," not a "downer." It is a stimulant, not an opiate. Walking, if done at a brisk rate (3 to 4 mph), stimulates the central nervous system and has an energizing effect, so you will have more energy after walking, not less.

Q: Will walking aggravate my varicose veins or cause blood clots?

A: The act of walking will not aggravate varicose veins or cause blood clots. Your major concern should be not with walking itself but with the precautions that you should be aware of after walking. Because blood tends to pool in the lower extremeties after you complete your walk, you should follow proper cool-down procedures (described later in this book) and should elevate your legs above your waist and massage them gently. Not only will your condition not deteriorate, it just might improve!

Q: Does walking elevate the blood pressure?

A: In the initial phases of walking, as is true with other forms of exercise, the blood pressure may become slightly elevated. However, a moderate walking program, introduced gradually, does not usually elevate the pressure of the blood to a dangerous level. If you have a tendency toward high blood pressure, dynamic strength exercises are the main exercises that should be avoided, not walking. In fact, the exercise prescription for hypertension recommended by most physicians is walking.

Q: Will going for a walk every day increase my life span?

A: Walking has been called an "anti-aging antibiotic," and I refer to it as "a drink from the fountain of youth," but walking has not been shown to have properties that will prolong life per se. At the same time, there is growing evidence that walking and other forms of continuous activity can arrest physical deterioration and reverse physical aging. The evidence is inconclusive as to whether walking will add years to your life, but I can state unequivocally that walking will add life to your years!

Q: Can I attain the "runner's high" by walking?

A: No, you cannot attain a "runner's high" from walking, but you can attain a "walker's high" from walking that is just as intense and overwhelming as any feeling that I have experienced. Each morning while I am walking and after I finish walking I feel good. Several times a week I feel intensely good. And once every two weeks or so, I reach a euphoric state as I go with the flow of my body. As I hit my stride, my movements become synchronized and I feel as if I am in a suspended state, walking on air, floating, soaring like a bird and feeling joyful, elated, and free. You, too, will experience that exhilarating feeling . . . just go with the flow.

Q: My enthusiasm for every exercise program that I have joined is short-lived. Why can't I stick with it?

A: Given such limited information and the fact that there are so many ways that the question can be interpreted, it's difficult for me to give you a definitive answer. Nevertheless, I will answer your question from an internal and external frame of reference and see if I can touch on what it is you have in mind.

From an internal perspective, you are saying, "I don't have any self-control, discipline, or willpower." Several behavioral researchers have suggested that it is helpful to view self-control as multidimensional and not as a single entity. In addition, self-control is not black or white and is not something that you have or don't have. You do have some self-control and you exert it every day in many areas. Therefore I suggest that you analyze your self-control in other areas and see if it can be transferred to the next time you start an exercise program. Second, try to come up with a reward that you can give yourself when you do exercise self-control in that program.

From the external perspective, you may be alluding to the fact that your environment is not always set up in a way to keep you interested. The exercise program you burned out on may have been boring, your expectations may have been unrealistic because you set your goals too high, the reinforcement from your family and friends might not have been strong enough, or the benefits may not have been easily recognized by you. The answer to your question is probably a combination of all of the above.

Q: Is it better to walk very briskly for a short distance or to walk at a moderate pace for a long distance?

A: That is like asking which came first, the chicken or the egg. Without begging the question, however, I must say that it depends on why you are going for a walk. If you are interested in receiving the cardiovascular benefits associated with walking, you must walk at a pace that is brisk enough to elevate your heart rate and sustain it at that level for 20 to 30 minutes. If, however, your reason for walking fast is to get it over with, then you are sacrificing enjoyment for speed, which is something that I bitterly oppose. The initial benefit from long-distance walking is primarily to increase your endurance, and the cardiovascular benefits are second-ary. Then too, the distance, speed, and terrain must be considered. There is no systematic research to my knowledge that shows that starting out walking briskly and gradually increasing your distance is any better over the long haul than walking at a moderate pace for a long distance and gradually decreasing the time that it takes to walk that distance. I have talked with walkers who have used both methods with equal success. Thus, from a long-range perspective, I think it balances out. What would be most reinforcing for you is the main issue, not speed versus distance. Personally I favor the long-distance walks. Why? Because the journey is more exciting than the destination. In both instances, to achieve a high level of fitness from walking, you will have to progressively make more demands on your body.

Q: Should I increase the distance that I walk gradually or in spurts?

A: A basic element underlying most physical activity programs is GRADUALISM. If you start fast you may finish last . . . or not at all. The fast start orientation is, in part, based on the propensity for instant success, which is another reason why so many people drop out of exercise programs. Has this ever happened to you? You make a commitment to engage in an activity, purchase the necessary equipment and/or pay the necessary membership dues, overexert and injure yourself, and then discontinue the activity. It is not surprising then that closets and attics throughout America are filled with golf clubs, tennis rackets, bowling balls, jogging suits, and other sports equipment collecting dust. This need not be the case if you approach changing your sedentary life-style gradually. You don't want to overexert or injure yourself, and you want the internal you to catch up with the external you—which is another way of saying you want your body to adjust naturally to the new active person that is emerging. Finally, you want to make lasting changes, irrespective of how small they may be, that will endure and persist. For all these reasons, the gradual approach is best.

The above questions and answers were designed to clear up some of the misconceptions that exist about walking. As you continue reading and experiencing what walking is, you will find answers to other questions. Two obvious questions, however, have not been asked: When should I walk? Where should I walk? Perhaps the answers to these questions are so elementary that they are taken for granted. Whatever the case, it must be pointed out that when and where are related directly to the second and third basic elements in a walking program, CONSISTENCY and ENJOYMENT. These are two of the elements that will keep you walking after the novelty has worn off.

4

When to Walk

For me, the early morning hours are best year-round for walking, for several reasons. First, I believe in putting first things first, and walking is the first item on my agenda every day. I schedule my day around my walking and not my walking around my day. Second, the morning is compatible with my work schedule since I often work late in the evening. Third, the morning hours allow for a minimal number of distractions, which means I can concentrate on specific things. Some mornings I concentrate on elevating my heart rate to achieve the best possible fitness benefits; on other mornings, I focus on enjoying my surroundings—or my solitude. Finally, walking into daylight, seeing the sun rise every morning and being an active partner in the production of a new day, is an exhilarating experience.

Mothers and housewives often report that morning hours are good for their walks too—after getting the children off to school and their husbands off to work. They leave the household chores for later in the morning and intersperse their pleasant morning walks with their out-of-house chores like shopping and going to the bank. Taking a morning walk is also a good weight management strategy for those who are tempted to snack in the morning or eat the food their children left on their breakfast plates.

Have you ever gone for a walk at lunchtime? For many people who work outside the home, this is an ideal time.

Want to join them? Select a restaurant 4 to 6 blocks away from your work site; the round trip will equal approximately 1 mile. If you eat your lunch in the place where you work, excuse yourself 10 to 15 minutes before the end of your lunch period and go for a walk in or around the building, climbing several flights of stairs if possible. Or select one or two days a week when you skip lunch, take a couple of pieces of fruit with you, and go window shopping—or to a nearby park for a brisk walk. Since brisk walking is a stimulant, your noontime walk will not only decrease the desire for an afternoon nap but will increase your productivity over the next 4 hours as well. Give it a try a couple of days a week and see if you don't notice a difference.

Walk Break

How about a walk break instead of a coffee break? Sounds absurd? Not really, if you think about it. I can cite an example of a group of women who use their 15-minute break in the morning and afternoon to go for a walk.

I discovered them quite by accident one morning a year or so ago walking at a moderate pace near my office. I didn't think much about it the first time I saw them but then, a couple of days later, I saw another group of women walking at the same pace, again in the same neighborhood. Over the next few weeks, whenever I happened to be out at mid-morning or mid-afternoon, I saw two, three, or more women walking the same route at a moderate pace. My curiosity got the best of me so I stopped the group and asked if they were actually going for a walk. They said yes and added that, since they did not smoke or drink coffee, the 15-minute morning and afternoon break was an ideal time for them to take a walk to refresh themselves.

The building where these women work (I don't know how many are employed there or how many participate in the walking break) is located across the street from the Upper Room on Grand Avenue in Nashville. So, if you visit Nashville and take a tour of the city that stops at the Upper Room at mid-morning or mid-afternoon, don't be surprised if you see a group of women exiting for their walking break.

Evening, either before or after dinner, is preferred by others as the best walking time. A stroll after work can reduce some of the tension of the work day, and walking before dinner can reduce hunger pangs that frequently occur in the early evening hours. Emotional eaters whom I have helped lose weight also report that walking at this time is very helpful in controlling the urge to eat before dinner. Then after dinner, the tight, full feeling that sometimes makes you feel uncomfortable and sleepy can be alleviated with a walk of a mile or two at a moderate pace. After-dinner walking is also helpful in elevating the basal metabolism to assist in burning fat. Wait an hour or so after dinner, though, before walking at a more brisk pace.

Do you sometimes want to spend more time with your spouse or a particular friend but find that other things tend to get in the way? One couple I know had this problem and I am sure it is typical of many. Since both of them work and they have teenage children, their schedule is quite hectic. Between the telephone ringing, the radio, stereo, and television blaring, the children's friends visiting, and having to transport the children to various events—not to mention their own daily household chores—their time together was minimal. They solved the problem by scheduling an evening walk several times a week, which provided them with an opportunity to be alone and to talk about their days—and their lives—with each other.

Late evening and night walks can be very romantic. On your next date, instead of going to a lavish party or out to dinner, how about a light snack at home followed by a long walk, with some talking and lots of hand-holding? If you haven't tried it lately, you really should!

Thus there is a great deal of flexibility as to when you can go for a walk. Flexibility, though, was only one point I wanted to make. The second point, though perhaps less obvious, was CONSISTENCY, the second basic element of walking.

Your daily walk, whether it is a brisk morning walk, an afternoon walk to the neighborhood store at a moderate pace, or a late evening stroll, must remain at the top of your "do" list each day. To truly experience what walking is, you must incorporate it on a regular basis into your daily routine to the point where it is an integral and inseparable part of your new life-style.

One dedicated walker comes to mind who refused to let external events affect a consistent walking schedule she had established.

Alice, 47 years of age, entered my weight management program to lose 35 pounds. She was a registered dietician and was well-versed in the nutritional needs of the body, but she needed the structure of a program to get started and felt the need to become more physically active. She began a consistent after-dinner walking program with her husband and soon started having good results. Since she had just moved to a new section of the country, relatives began visiting. Although she entertained her relatives in a royal manner, she, along with her husband, refused to give up her evening walk. Instead of sitting around the table eating more after dinner, Alice invited the relatives to go for a walk. At first there were snickers and barbs, but over time the message got across and soon when the relatives returned home, they wrote or called to express thanks for the hospitality and for the walks—and some even indicated that they were building an evening walk into their own lives. Now the word is out in the family: If you go to visit Alice, you can plan in advance to go for a walk after dinner.

Alice's determination not only paid off for her but also influenced at least some members of her family. The message is clear: Plan your day around your walking and not your walking around your day. The consistent walker does not try to find time to go for a walk. The consistent walker makes time to go for a walk.

Ready for your second assignment?

Assignment: Develop a Walking Schedule

One way to approach finding the times that are best for you is by developing a walking schedule. Use the form on the next page to identify the best days and times for you to go for a walk. The first question you must ask yourself concerns your typical daily schedule. Select the least busy days of the week and list on the form all the activities that you engage in on those particular days. Put one asterisk (*) over those days. (Yes, I know that your routine varies from one week to the next, but you can surely find *some* common patterns.) Done? Good. Now pick the days that you are typically most busy and list all of the activities you engage in on those days. Put two asterisks (**) over those days.

Review your weekly schedule. Do you have a half-hour or an hour free on your least busy day or days when you can go for a walk? If so, put a W for WALKING in all of the spaces that would be compatible with going for a walk. How many entries were you able to make?

Now take another look. Do you have a half-hour or an hour on your busiest day or days when you can go for a walk? If so, yes, you guessed it. Put a W in those spaces.

If you have more than two days when you can walk at the same time, you are on your way to becoming a consistent walker. If you do not, is it possible to rearrange any part of your schedule or shift your priorities in such a way that you can walk during the same time period several days a week? The main idea is to arrange your life in such a way that you can walk at the same time every day, or on as many days as possible and feasible.

Once you have decided on your walking times, construct a walking schedule that you can place in a very conspicuous spot in your home. Family members will not have to worry about where you are or when you will return, and your walking schedule will indicate what you are doing . . . WALKING.

Best Days and Times for Walking

Hour	Sun	Mon	Tu	Wed	Th	Fri	Sat
7:00–8:00							
8:00–9:00							
9:00–10:00							
10:00–11:00							
11:00–12:00							
12:00–1:00							
1:00–2:00							
2:00–3:00							
3:00–4:00							
4:00–5:00							
5:00–6:00							
6:00–7:00							
7:00–8:00							
8:00–9:00							
9:00–10:00							
10:00–11:00							

5

Where to Walk

In deciding *when* to walk, you can choose the season, the month, the week, the day, the hour, even the minute. The *where* of walking, however, is limited to one of two choices: indoors or outdoors. Even though you may find that your preference for one over the other will change from day to day, as you begin to experience what walking is, you will probably enjoy both.

I will not attempt to provide you with an exhaustive list of indoor and outdoor places to walk, but I will point out some possibilities based on my knowledge of areas that have proved helpful to me and to others over the years. The main emphasis will be on getting you to use your imagination and creativity to find areas for walking that are best for you. Because I am concerned with making walking a pleasant experience, I want first to say a word or two about the third basic element in walking, ENJOYMENT. Later in the chapter I will also talk about safety precautions.

Enjoyment

In order for you to continue any physical activity after the novelty has worn off, it must be enjoyable. Exercise leaders may disagree on the necessary elements or on the ordering of the elements for a successful physical activity program, but most would agree that enjoyment is basic. Dr. George Sheehan, an inspirational force in the jogging movement, calls it play. He began jogging at the age of 44 and said he discovered play. Dr. Art Ulene, in his book *Feeling Fine*, called it fun—exercising and "feeling fine" is fun. In addition, many coaches feel that enjoyment of a particular sport is critical to maximal performance. Joe Paterno, when interviewed on "60 Minutes" prior to the 1979 Cotton Bowl game, said it best:

> The boys work hard all week in practice; therefore, Saturday should be fun—win, lose, or draw. If playing on Saturday is not fun, what is the purpose of practicing all week?

Professional athletes have also recognized the importance of enjoying participating in a sport when deciding to retire. In their retirement speeches, the message is usually the same:

> I don't enjoy training and practicing. The game isn't fun anymore.

Although many professional athletes receive large annual salaries for participating in a sport for 6 months or less out of the year, money alone is apparently not enough. The game has to be enjoyable for them to perform day after day during the season for a number of years. The same attitude applies to walking. If it isn't fun, it will soon become boring and you will lose interest in it. You will not give your best, and in fact, you will gradually begin to find excuses and will eventually discontinue it.

So how do you make walking a fun thing—a form of play—an enjoyable experience? Each of you will find your own way, but read on and I'll share with you some of the reasons walking continues to be pleasurable for me and a number of other walking enthusiasts.

Indoor Walking

What are the criteria for selecting an indoor walking place? It turns out that just about any indoor area that is spacious enough for continuous walking and that will not

bore you is adequate. First, start with your home or apartment and take an inventory of the space inside. Is it spacious
enough for a 5- or 10-minute walk? If your answer is no, I
would like for you to reconsider the question. For instance,
how long would you walk if you started in the basement,
walked around the perimeter of each room, walked upstairs
to the first floor and walked around the perimeter of each
room and then walked around the perimeter of each room
on the next floor? If you have space on only one floor, how
long would it take you to walk the perimeter of that space
twice in one direction and then twice in the other direction?
One dedicated walker who spent 2 weeks inside her home
during a heavy snowfall last year told me that she got in her
2 miles of walking each day by going through the house 27
times without stopping.

The assessment of your neighborhood is the next step. Is
there a building within a 4-block radius where you can walk
indoors continuously? Are there also buildings within an 8-
or 12-block radius? Take a moment and think about it and
see if you can identify several buildings in your area that
would be appropriate for indoor walking.

Two good indoor walking places are hotels and shopping
malls. At a recent convention in Atlanta, several of my colleagues who were joggers had not brought their jogging
attire so I invited them to accompany me on a walk through
the hotel. The walk consisted of climbing each flight of stairs
and walking down around the hall of each floor between
flights. The walk to the 27th floor took approximately 35
minutes and I calculated that we had walked 3 miles.

Shopping malls in the early morning hours before the
stores open are especially appealing to walkers. In the Nashville area, three shopping malls give walkers special consideration and allow cardiac patients, the elderly, and others to
walk in the mall before the regular opening time. Some
merchants have gone so far as to place attendance books in
their stores for walkers to enter the number of miles walked
each day. Check out the malls in your area. The odds are 3

to 1 that you will find some happy walkers there 5 days a week.

Another good place for indoor walking is a large hospital or a university medical center. Have you ever tried to find a particular clinic in a hospital, turned left instead of right, and ended up having to walk a quarter of a mile to reach your original destination? Think how much better you would have felt if you had taken that "wrong" turn intentionally! Most medical center complexes also contain underground tunnels and interlocking buildings that are appropriate for continuous walking.

The next time you visit a friend or family member in the hospital, stop by the information desk, pick up a map, and go for a walk around the hospital first. That quarter- or half-mile walk before you enter the room could make the difference between a pleasant, cheerful visit and a depressing one. After your visit, take another brief walk before you leave the hospital and focus on the positive things that occurred during your stay.

If you are employed, is there a long corridor near your work area where you can walk back and forth several times for 10 or 15 minutes at a time? Does your building have more than two stories? If so, can you walk up several flights of stairs, and then walk down the corridor and back down several flights of stairs? What about the basement and the area where the supplies are kept?

The halls of schools are excellent for sustained walking, as exemplified by the following description of a committed walker.

Kim, a school teacher, had gained 10 pounds over the holidays and was concerned about the tightness of her clothes. She began arriving at school a half hour before her classes started and going for a 1- or 2-mile brisk walk down the long and winding corridors of the large comprehensive high school. She meticulously measured out her walking course and soon enlisted other teachers to walk with her. Her diet was not altered but she walked in the morning at school and then stopped off at a local park after school to walk an additional 2 to 3 miles. She also increased her walking on the weekends. Her rationale was simple: "I eat more on the weekend, so I walk more on the weekend." In 4 months, she reached her ideal weight, and became committed to daily brisk walking. Walking became a positive addiction. She started a walk-jog program, began jogging 3 to 4 miles every day, and eventually participated in the local Bonne Bell Race (6.2 miles), in which she finished Number 349 out of 800 participants, her first time out.

Is it possible for you to use the school or the gymnasium in your community for walking? What would happen if you approached the local school board and asked them to open the building an hour earlier than usual 2 days each week for walkers? This notion may not be as far-out as it sounds. By increasing the visibility of parents as physically active role models, this notion could have a significant impact on the children, the school system, the community, the state, and the nation. Walking can also be seen as patriotic, since a strong America is extricably tied to the physical fitness of our children.

The major objection to indoor walking is that it is boring, but for a growing number of walkers, the advantages that it offers outweigh the disadvantages. For instance, indoor walking is usually convenient, it helps you develop consistency, it can add variety to your daily walk, and, in most instances, it is safe. In addition, you will never have to wonder where you will walk when inclement weather occurs. You will have already identified several indoor sites that can be used to keep you on your daily schedule. Is indoor walking for you? Read the section on outdoor walking before you decide.

Outdoor Walking

Open your front door and survey your neighborhood. You will see that a walking path exists all around you. If you are going for a brisk walk, walking where you have to pause at a stop light or wait for traffic every block or so is very discouraging. Therefore, search for an area where you can walk continuously with a minimal number of stops. Take a personal inventory of the 4-block radius, 8-block radius, and 12-block radius as you did in finding a place for indoor walking. But this time, select areas where you can walk uninterrupted for 15 to 20 minutes. Use a street map of your area to identify several good walking sites. For continuous walking, the following outdoor sites are recommended: perimeters of elementary and high schools, large parking lots of churches, country roads, and main thoroughfares near your neighborhood. Don't forget, either, about high school and college tracks.

Residents in the Nashville area were recently informed that nine high school tracks were available for walking at night and that information on the location of light switches for each track could be obtained from the principal or from the Board of Education. Perhaps similar provisions have been made in your community?

What about public parks in your area? They are ideal for a relaxing stroll and, at certain times of the day and season, they are very appropriate for brisk walking. You are urged, however, to experiment, to be creative, and to use your imagination to find the walking path that is best for you.

I have lots more to say, but right now I want to experience the pleasure of walking instead of writing about it. Won't you join me?

On Becoming a Walking Explorer

Experimentation and exploration may add a new and different dimension to your walking experience—at least that is what happens to me as I seek out new areas for pleasurable walking. Thus I walk in as many places as possible. I like variety. Most of the time, my exploration is planned, but then on occasion, if time permits, I take off on an unplanned expedition.

My favorite place for planned exploration is college campuses, and my favorite day and time is on Sunday morning. In the Nashville area, there are many beautiful campuses, and once a month I select one and stroll by the buildings, fantasizing about the architectural structure, purpose of the buildings, and occupants of the buildings. On the campus of David Lipscomb College in Nashville, there is a bronze statue of a bison near the tennis court. I stop momentarily and touch the statue and wonder about its significance to the college. As I walk on the campus of Frisk University and pass Jubilee Hall and the chapel where the Jubilee Singers raised their voices in song many years ago, I wonder if the musical tradition still exists. On the Peabody College campus of Vanderbilt University there is a Kennedy Center, and a quarter of a mile away, a Social-Religious Building. What function do these buildings serve? Is the Kennedy Center associated with the Kennedy family? Elsewhere on the Vanderbilt campus there is a massive statue of Charles Sarratt casting an imposing shadow across the campus in the early morning hours. Who was Sarratt and what role did he play in the development of the university?

When I go outside Nashville, my exploration of college campuses continues. As I walk the midway adjacent to the University of Chicago, starting at Cottage Grove Avenue, walking East on 58th and passing the large hospital complex and the English building, I wonder if Saul Bellow is inside busily writing a sequel to his famous novel, *Herzog*. I can then take a half-mile detour and go past Stagg Field and read the plaque commemorating the spot where the atom was broken in 1941—or continue walking eastward and pass the famous Rockefeller Chapel. I enjoy the McKendree College campus in Lebanon, Illinois, walking past Old Main and the historic chapel. Also the University of Illinois at Urbana-Champaign, from Illini Hall to the dome-shaped assembly hall 2 miles away. Atlanta University Center includes five colleges—Morehouse, Spellman, Clark, Morris Brown, and the Baptist Institute—all of which are located within the same general area where it is possible to cross the street and go from one campus to the other. American University in Washington, D.C., the Bronx campus of New York University, and Denver University in the Mile High City are just a few of the campuses where I have gone for interesting and instructive walks. It is such an enjoyable activity that I hope to walk on every major college campus in America before the year 2000.

I feel a certain serenity as I walk on a college campus in the early morning hours. The students are sleeping late from their hours of studying or partying, and I have the campus to myself, with just the trees, birds, and squirrels. Occasionally, I stop to read a cornerstone or look at the tall columns of a building to see if they are Ionic or Doric and to figure out the period of time that influenced the structure of the building.

At your earliest opportunity, get a map of the college in your community and take a walking tour of the campus. Or, if you really want to become stimulated while walking, just explore the campus on your own. Search for the adventurer in yourself and fantasize as you explore.

Nature Walks: A Special Treat

Up to this point, I have talked about walking in the city, and have suggested a number of places that you might enjoy going for a walk. But perhaps you do not live in the city, and maybe you do not live near a college campus. That should not stop you from finding an exciting place to experience the joy of walking. In fact, if you live in the suburbs, in a small town, or on a farm, you just may have a distinct advantage over the urban dweller. Your sparsely populated area with less traffic and tranquil surroundings is quite conducive to walking.

Even though I enjoy walking along the busy boulevards in the city, or finding indoor places to walk for variety, or

planned and unplanned explorations, I sometimes find myself compelled to head for the forest to get closer to man's
natural habitat. Is it because of boredom with the city streets
and buildings? The need to find a more tranquil setting? The
need to mimic the great walkers of old? Whatever the reason, I find a need to retreat from the urban setting to walk
with nature. I search for the peace and serenity that can only
be found walking in the woods and forest, where the peck-
ing order has been established and the natural flow of survival has gone on for years.

Eighteenth- and nineteenth-century writers seem to have
discovered the importance of nature walks before me, as
reflected in the writings I mentioned earlier of Frost, Whitman, Thoreau, Carlyle, and Wordsworth. When someone
asked Wordsworth's secretary for a tour of his working area,
she remarked, "This is his library, but he works out of doors
while walking." This orientation has carried over to many
modern-day writers, who are often quoted as saying that
they retreat to a cabin in the woods to develop their
thoughts about a novel.

One contemporary naturalist, Edwin Teal, had a distinct
advantage in that he lived with nature constantly. He wrote
a book entitled *A Walk Through the Years* that was a diary of
his walking experiences for one year. Teal's description of
each daily walk was vivid and revealing. For instance, on
describing one of his walks, he showed how much in touch
he was with his surroundings:

> Without thinking what I am doing, without conscious effort of
> observation, I drink in the sights and sounds and smells I find
> around me. It is so that I walk through the woods today.

In his diary, he recorded the ushering in and out of the four
seasons and the profound effect that it had on him as he
walked through the woods each day.

Walking in the natural elements has always fascinated
man, and several years ago a professor at Franklin Pierce
College in New Hampshire offered a course that consisted

of a long walk during the semester. The major rationale for offering such a course? In the professor's words:

> In school again, I found it difficult to stick to the subject. I wanted to talk about the world now . . . our lives. My only excuse was that I was burning to get out of books and plays and research and into our whole lives; physical, emotional, and intellectual.

The walking project involved walking 550 miles from the campus of the school to Halifax, Nova Scotia, averaging 15 miles a day. The book, entitled *The Walk of the Conscious Ants,* was dedicated to all the students enrolled in the course. Their classroom was the open road and their textbook was America. During the process of taking a college course, Philosophy of Walking, they discovered the joy of awakening under a canopy of pine branches, the power of an old-time revival meeting, and the excitement of a ladies' wrestling match. They discovered America in a new and unique way.

Walking with nature in any season gives us the opportunity to capture the best of both worlds: pure enjoyment and the return to our roots. The peace and serenity of the woods offers a calming and soothing effect that cannot be found anyplace else—including the therapist's couch. Nature walking is one way of our prescribing what is best for ourselves. Through the medium of writing, different individuals have recorded words to preserve our history and have used walking as a vehicle. However, without a pen, we can pick our season and record it indelibly in our minds by using our eyes as a permanent camera and the inner resources of our mind to recall an unforgettable stroll.

Safety Precautions

Walking has been presented as an activity that is for the famous as well as the nonfamous, that is for the aging as well as for the young, that is ideal anytime and anyplace, and that is an activity that can be easily fit into your present life-style. All of this is true, but there is another side of the coin. For instance, what do you do if you are afraid of dogs? How do you handle a ferocious one? How do you distinguish a friendly bark from a dangerous growl? How do you handle a molester or would-be robber? These are questions that are asked frequently by new walkers and that are cited as the reason for not starting a walking program or for discontinuing one—but this need not be the case.

I must admit to you that I am neither a professional dog handler adept in the techniques of making ferocious dogs friendly nor a 7th degree Black Belt who is proficient in martial arts techniques to ward off robbers. While these qualifications might be helpful in certain situations, I do feel qualified to assure you that they are not essential for pleasurable walking.

I have listed below some strategies and procedures that will facilitate your walking if you have anxious moments when the neighborhood dog charges toward you or a suspicious stranger approaches. About dogs:

Do	Don't
Ignore the dog	Show that you are afraid
Continue walking briskly and with confidence	Run from the dog
Walk with a friend or in a group	Intimidate the dog except to tell it to go home
Stop and tell the dog to go home in a firm voice if the dog pursues you	Pet the dog
Check the leash law and call the owner and/or appropriate officials	Throw objects at the dog
	Give up walking

As you begin to walk a particular route, the neighborhood dogs will get to know you, will bark less, and in time will ignore you. More than anything else, the dogs are reacting to a stranger walking in their neighborhood, which is a normal reaction. After a few days of walking the same route, you will not be a stranger and they will begin ignoring you —or joining you proudly for a walk of their own. Do you remember reading earlier about the second basic element, CONSISTENCY? This is one of those places where it will really pay off for you.

Here is a list of tips that you might try to reduce the chances of flirtatious advances and to handle would-be molesters and robbers:

Do	Don't
Leave your purse, money, and valuables at home or locked in the trunk of your car	Carry a purse
	Walk alone in isolated and deserted areas
If possible, walk on a main thoroughfare	Walk alone at night
	Wear provocative clothing
Occasionally vary the time and day when you walk	Stop and talk to strangers
	Overreact—but be alert
Vary your walking route	Give up walking
Carry an umbrella or walking stick	
Walk briskly and with confidence	

Sudden thundershowers, going to the bathroom, responding to emergencies, and other matters are additional concerns. Here are a few more safety precautions:

Do	Don't
Carry a piece of identification	Drink coffee or other liquids before walking if you have a weak bladder
Carry small change for an emergency telephone call	Continue walking if you become ill
Check the weather report	Take refuge under a tree when there is lightning
Go to the bathroom before leaving the house	Walk briskly at night on a rocky surface or where there are potholes
Wear light-colored clothing to reflect the light at night	Walk against a red light just to keep up your pace
Walk facing the traffic on roads that are narrow	Give up walking
Let your family or a friend know your walking route and when you expect to return	
Call the police if you feel you are being followed and/or if you notice strange cars parked in or cruising the area	

TIME-OUT

I feel the need here, since I cannot personally walk with you every step of the way, for a TIME-OUT. The reason for this is twofold: to ascertain if you have indeed gotten started on the right foot, and to see if you are ready for additional information to keep you going. So, at this critical juncture, I would like for you to stop for a moment to take an inventory and answer the following questions.

Have you been reading and doing? Did you go for the leisurely stroll that I recommended? Did you assess it afterward by answering the questions? Did you complete the assignment on developing a walking schedule? Have you found a safe place to go for a walk? Are you making time to go for a walk every day? If you responded no to all of these questions, you have missed a vital part of the walking experience.

What I have presented thus far is a personal approach to experiencing what walking is. This approach will work for you if you get in step and give it a chance. However, with persons from various age groups and different levels of fitness reading this book, it is natural to expect a slight nudge from some of you concerning the pace. I am aware of the broad continuum of knowledge and interest that you represent, so I welcome your nudge.

I am sure some of you are interested in moving faster. Others are satisfied with the pace. Still others would like to slow the pace. There is no timetable for reading or finishing this book. YOU can decide when and if you are ready for a change of pace. Be honest with yourself as you continue taking your inventory.

Am I moving too fast? Is there an information overload? Do you get the feeling that you are being bombarded with a lot of new information before you have had an opportunity to try out some of the old suggestions? Do you prefer to take things one step at a time and feel comfortable with one area before proceeding to another? My advice to you is to do less reading and more walking. If you feel the need to re-read one or all of the chapters, or to wait a week or two before reading further, fine.

What about those of you who are interested in moving faster? Are you bored with the assignments? Do you find the reports about successful walkers simplistic and uninspiring? Are you ready for more structure? Are you ready for a walking program that gets right to the heart of the matter? Then I recommend that you read the sections on shoes and wearing apparel in the next chapter and then skip to the program at the back of the book.

Do some of you feel that the pace is right on target? If you are following the basic principles of GRADUALISM, CONSISTENCY, and ENJOYMENT, fantastic! Don't rock the boat if you are experiencing the joy of walking at your present pace.

How about the assignments? If you have not done them, I strongly urge you to go back and do them now. The longer you postpone them, the less meaningful they will be to you. Of course whether you even do them—or increase or decrease your "read and do pace"—or let this book collect dust on your living room table—all are decisions that only you can make.

Are you resisting my suggestion because you think you will lose your momentum? Then let me be a bit philosophical about it: A slight detour and a brief respite of a couple of days are a small sacrifice to make to build the foundation for a walking experience that may last a lifetime. It is not too late to get in step and experience the joy of walking.

YOU HAVE A CHOICE.
NOW IS THE TIME TO EXERCISE IT!

6

Walking Aids

Even though you have probably made significant strides since you began experiencing what walking is, I want to caution you against becoming overly confident and thinking that you are ready to go it alone. Perhaps you are ready, but I doubt it! You did not become sedentary overnight and you are not going to become a serious and committed walker in a few weeks. I am not saying this to dampen your enthusiasm, but simply to point out the difficulties many people have in maintaining their motivation after the novelty of walking has worn off. That is why it is important today, not tomorrow, to begin developing a new mind set that has as its central focus keeping you walking and preventing a relapse. There are certain preventive measures that will reduce the likelihood of a relapse, but when one does occur (and it will!) I want you to be prepared to make it a temporary one. One way to prepare yourself is with an armamentarium of aids.

By definition, *aid* refers to that which is useful or necessary in achieving an end. Broadly speaking, then, there are many categories of aids. For one, there are aids in the form of equipment and instruments that are designed to ensure comfort and/or assist in mobility as in the case of shoes and other wearing apparel. Second, there are aids in the form of strategies and techniques that are used to help assist in achieving long-term goals. While it may appear that shoes and strategies being classified together are a poor fit, they do, in fact, go together quite well. Both are necessary and useful and will help you achieve an objective. Both will make walking a more meaningful and enjoyable experience. Both will keep you going.

In the early part of this chapter, then, I will talk about an aid that is basic and necessary, namely, good shoes, and then later in the chapter I will talk about wearing apparel and strategies such as charts and maps that I, along with other walkers, have found to be useful in preventing relapses.

Shoes

A distinct advantage that walkers have over joggers, tennis buffs, golfers, and other sports enthusiasts is simplicity in attire. There is no need to go out and purchase a special wardrobe. With the exception of shoes, you are likely to find all of the apparel needed right in your own closet in order for you to become a full-fledged member of the silent majority. Shoes, the most important piece of equipment for walking, are another matter and deserve careful consideration.

In general, any shoe that is comfortable and feels good can be used for walking. If, based on the amount of walking you are doing, your present shoes fit this criterion and you are not experiencing any difficulty, continue wearing them. On the other hand, if you are in the market for a new pair of shoes or you suspect that the ones you are wearing are inappropriate, read this section carefully.

There are a number of popular and lesser known brand names of walking shoes that are appropriate for sauntering or brisk walking. Rather than tell you which brand to buy or not to buy, I will outline an approach to evaluating and purchasing a walking shoe. The onus will then be on you to make your own selection.

Why Should You Be Concerned with a Walking Shoe?

Given the fact that you are going to walk hundreds of miles during the coming months, you need shoes that will add pleasure, maximize comfort, and minimize the possibility of injury.

WHAT Are the Characteristics of a Good Walking Shoe?

One of the important characteristics of a walking shoe is a snug fit. A walking shoe should fit snug like a glove at the heel and the instep and should conform to the natural outline of your foot. The longest toe should be ½ to 1 inch from the front of the shoe and you should be able to lift, wiggle, and spread your toes without difficulty.

A second characteristic of a good walking shoe is heel support. The heel strikes the walking surface innumerable times in your lifetime, as illustrated in computations that appear later in this book. Thus it is important that the heel be broad enough to provide adequate support to absorb the impact of the weight of your body. The heel of your walking shoe should be elevated ½ to ¾ inches higher than the sole to relieve the strain on the back of the leg. Most walking and jogging shoes have a double or triple layered heel to absorb the impact of each step and a waffled or treaded sole and heel to assure adequate traction for your heel when it strikes the walking surface—and for pushing off with your toes. High heels tend to throw the body out of line and exert pressure on your toes and instep, and smooth soles without heels (including tennis shoes) tend to exert pressure on the achilles tendon. Neither type of shoe is usually suitable for sustained walking.

Inner lining, arch supports, and obstructions are other characteristics that need to be considered. The inner padding for the sole and heel should be soft and spongy to absorb the impact of walking, but the padding should be a little rough to adhere to your socks so that your feet do not slide too far down in the shoes. Flex your toes and move them around to see if any portion of the upper lining touches your toes. A slight obstruction or rubbing against the toes in this area will become pronounced as you begin wearing the shoes. If you feel an obstruction inside the shoe, it might be because of the stitching across the outside of the shoe. Look at the stitching and connecting points on the outside of the shoe and see if this stitching is cutting across any of your toes.

Most walking shoes are constructed with a soft absorbent padding that conforms to the arch of the foot. This, however, is not an arch support, so if you have a history of fallen arches or if you are prone to injuries in this area of your foot, a worthwhile investment would be for you to see a podiatrist and have a special arch support constructed for your foot that can be transferred from shoe to shoe.

How about pliability? Does the shoe bend easily at the top third of the shoe? Durability . . . does it appear that the shoe can handle the terrain in your area of the country? Breathability . . . does the shoe breathe and allow proper aeration and ventilation? These are also important characteristics in the selection of a walking shoe.

WHEN Do You Purchase a Walking Shoe?

When refers not only to the time of day for purchasing your shoes, but also that point at which old shoes should be discarded and a new pair purchased. As far as the time of day is concerned, I recommend that shoes be purchased in the afternoon or early evening since your feet swell during the day. A shoe that fits perfectly in the morning may feel tight and constricted in the afternoon and at night. Old shoes are not appropriate for sustained walking when the sole and ball of the shoe become bald or slick or when you can begin feeling the walking surface through the shoe. In addition, when the heel is worn over to the point where you can feel your ankle turning outward when your heel touches the walking surface, the shoes should be retired. Worn-over heels and bald soles can lead to slips and falls, due to the loss of traction, and may precipitate injuries such as damage to your ankles or achilles tendons.

WHERE Do You Purchase a Walking Shoe?

Sporting goods stores and other businesses that cater to the needs of walkers and joggers are the most appropriate places to shop for walking shoes. Many of these stores sell jogging shoes, hiking boots, and leather walking shoes. Department stores usually have a more extensive line of leather walking shoes, but the personnel tend to be more concerned with style and a sale than with your comfort and safety. Therefore, if necessary, inform the salesperson that you will be walking 3 to 7 miles per day and that you want to purchase a walking shoe that will sustain you through that kind of program. The price range for a jogging shoe or a leather walking shoe is $45 to $65. Both are appropriate for sustained walking.

When you are in the market for your second pair of walking shoes, shop around the sporting goods stores for a sale. Most of these stores will have a sale on popular brand shoes several times a year. Leave your name and telephone number with a salesperson and ask him/her to call you the next time the store is having a sale on walking shoes. You will be able to save yourself $5 to $10 at least.

Do not purchase walking shoes through the mail or let someone else purchase them for you. You need to try them on before you buy them. Then, too, the process of returning the shoes might take 2 to 3 weeks—weeks in which you could have been out walking!

HOW Do You Purchase a Walking Shoe?

The cardinal rule in purchasing walking shoes is that function precedes fashion. To put it another way, your immediate concern is comfort, pliability, breathability, and durability. If the shoe looks good too, that is a bonus.

On entering a store to purchase a walking shoe, take 5 to

10 minutes to browse around the store and ask questions about the different shoes before you sit down. Pick up several pairs of shoes and look them over thoroughly. Turn them over and examine the heel and sole. Run your hand inside and feel the lining, the arch support, and the areas where your toes will be located. Bend the shoe to see if it is flexible. Now you are ready to try on shoes. Not one pair, but several pairs.

Ask the salesperson to measure your right and left foot. To your surprise, perhaps, you will probably discover that one foot is slightly larger than the other. Always try the shoe on the larger foot first. Tell the salesperson the purpose of the shoes if you have not already done so. You are now ready to begin a serious process of elimination and selection. I reiterate: Good walking shoes are the most important equipment you will purchase for walking. Take your time and select the best walking shoe for your particular feet. Be prepared to go to a number of stores if necessary.

After inspecting several pairs of shoes, having your feet measured and being fitted with both shoes, stand up in the shoes, wiggle your toes, check the fit of the heel, check the pliability, and then go for a walk around the store. Walk back and forth in front of a mirror.

Shoes that feel perfect while walking on the carpet inside the store will feel different when you walk on a hard surface. Ask the salesperson if you could try them out "in the real world" by going for a walk around the block. (In a department store, such a request might be met with astonishment, and possibly even an invitation to take a very long walk indeed, but you may be pleasantly surprised at the response you receive in a sporting goods store—especially one that caters to walkers and joggers.)

On re-entering the store, look in the mirror again and check for appearance. Do the shoes do anything for you? Are they your favorite color? If not, can you get the same shoes in another color? Most important, do the shoes make you feel and look like a walker?

Ask the salesperson about the maintenance and care of the shoes. Are there any special precautions that need to be taken? Tennis shoes can usually be machine washed and dried, but this is generally not the case with jogging and walking shoes. Jogging and walking shoes are usually hand-washed or cleaned with a special cleanser and air dried.

Should the new shoes be worn all day? It is usually recommended that you break your shoes in gradually by wearing them around the house. Then go for a short walk for several days before walking extensively in them.

Leather Shoes

Although jogging shoes are appropriate for walking in cold weather for up to an hour, you might be interested in leather walking shoes or hiking boots if you live in a really cold climate. When buying leather shoes, make sure they are pliable and durable. A good leather shoe will mold itself to the upper structure of the foot, will breathe and allow fresh air to circulate and cool your feet, and will simultaneously allow perspiration to evaporate.

I have several pairs of shoes and I match their use to the why and where of walking. I have cleated hiking boots that are waterproofed for excursions in the woods, for hiking trails, and for walking in the snow. I have jogging shoes that I use for 8- to 10-mile walks, and I have leather walking shoes for long-distance winter walking. My philosophy on shoes is that basketball shoes are for playing basketball, tennis shoes are for playing tennis, jogging shoes are for jogging (although they are interchangeable to some extent with walking shoes), high heels are for dressing stylishly, flats are for dancers and ballerinas, and walking shoes are for walking.

Assignment: Buy a Pair of Good Walking Shoes

This assignment, which is optional if you already have a good pair, is for you to purchase a pair of comfortable walking shoes. Do not take this assignment lightly. You will be making an investment of your time and your money for a basic walking aid that will add immeasurably to your comfort, safety, and happiness. As I stated earlier, a few extra minutes, or even days for that matter, of shopping for the shoes that are best for you will pay off handsomely several months from now.

Ask yourself the following important questions as you shop for your new walking shoes.

Does this shoe fit snug like a glove?	yes no
Does my heel fit snugly into the heel cup of the shoe?	yes no
Is the heel rim biting into my achilles tendon with each step?	yes no
Is there slippage of my heel?	yes no
Is my foot sliding down too much when I walk in the shoe?	yes no
Can I flex my toes?	yes no
Is there an obstruction which my toe keeps hitting?	yes no
Does the arch support feel right?	yes no
Does the shoe feel light?	yes no
Is the heel wide enough to absorb the impact?	yes no
Do the shoes make me feel and look like a walker?	yes no
Is this a good investment?	yes no

(If the answer to the previous question was yes, then the answer to this one is yes)

Socks

Whether you purchase your socks at the same store or not, always ask about the most appropriate socks to wear for walking in the shoes that you are about to buy. Socks should fit like shoes—snugly, with room enough for flexing your toes. Socks should be seamless, especially in chafe prone areas like the heels and balls of your feet. They should fit the contour of your foot. Heavy wool socks or two pairs of lighter socks are often worn by hikers and long distance walkers, but they are not needed for daily brisk walking. Socks made from natural products (light wool and cotton) which breathe, absorb perspiration, provide a good fit, and do not move around on the foot are recommended. Socks that are too small or too large can be as much of a problem as shoes that are too small or too large. Tight socks constrict the blood vessels in the foot, and loose socks that slide about on your foot as you are walking can contribute to the formation of blisters.

Smooth out any folds from the bottom of your foot and press the sock firmly against each foot before putting on your shoe. On a long walk, a folded sock can be as irritating as a rock in your shoe—and almost as damaging.

Hats

If you perspire heavily during the summer, you might want to consider a terrycloth head band or a straw hat to reflect the sun and keep your head cool. During the winter months, reducing the dissipation of heat from your head is a prime concern since approximately 40% of your body heat is lost through your head.

Wear a head scarf or a cotton stocking cap to prevent heat loss. In addition, the stocking cap can be pulled down over your ears if they get cold. A wool stocking cap should be reserved for colder temperatures, as well as earmuffs and a ski mask to protect the face and ears from frostbite.

Gloves

Another area of the body that loses heat is the fingertips, which are also particularly susceptible to frostbite. Gloves should be worn when the temperature dips below 45 degrees. A pair of cotton gardening gloves or work gloves that allow adequate warmth and ventilation are appropriate and inexpensive. Wool gloves and fur-lined gloves should be worn after the temperature drops to 20 degrees or below, especially if your hands are sensitive to colder temperatures.

General Attire

As a general rule, your attire for walking should be comfortable, practical, and minimal. During the spring and summer months, light-colored garments to reflect the sun and loose-fitting clothing that allows adequate ventilation are recommended. Bermuda shorts, walking shorts, culottes, pants, skirts and blouses, dresses, T-shirts, and tank tops are all ideal attire.

In the fall and winter months, dress in layers according to the temperature. A short-sleeved or long-sleeved cotton shirt or blouse, a pair of cotton trousers, and a light windbreaker or sweater will suffice in most areas of the country in the fall. Since the body warms up as you walk, you do not want to overdress. Heavy jackets or coats will cause you to perspire after walking several blocks, especially if you are walking at a brisk pace. Thermal underwear, leotards, or an extra pair of pantyhose are recommended in colder climates, but the undergarments should not be so tight they interfere with the natural flow of walking. You can unbutton your shirt or remove your jacket as you feel yourself becoming overheated, but personal discretion dictates that you keep your thermal underwear on until you get home.

In sum, then, a good pair of walking shoes is basic to ensuring your comfort and reducing the possibilities of injury. Beyond that, there are very few rules about what you can or should wear except the general rule that less is best. It is a matter of personal taste.

Walking Sticks

The walking stick has aided man in a number of ways down through the ages . . . as a device to conceal a blade or a knife, as a flask to hold alcoholic beverages, and as a means of support and stability for aging members of the population, to name a few.

Today there is a resurgence of interest in the walking stick for style, but for the serious walker who is experiencing the joys of walking, there are additional advantages. For one, it is a good defensive weapon that can be used to ward off potential muggers. A mugger will think twice before attacking when you are walking briskly with a walking stick.

Second, a walking stick can be used as an exercise aid. I am referring to "mini" exercises that you can incorporate while walking to increase your range of motion and improve your coordination. When I talk about warm-up and cool-down exercises in the Walking Program at the back of the book, I will recommend specific stretching exercises that you can approach in a more systematic way. For now, be creative and spontaneous. On your next walk, take your walking stick, raise it over your head with both hands, and push upward. Then, with the stick held high overhead, lean slowly to one side, then to the other. Toss the stick from one hand to the other as you walk. When you are waiting for a traffic light to turn green, use that brief interval to increase your wrist and finger dexterity by twirling your walking stick like a baton, first with the left hand and then with the right. Oops! You dropped it—but that's OK. With your knees locked, reach upward as far as possible, then slowly bend over and let your body hang and see if you can pick it up. You can't? That's OK too. You have just given your hamstring muscles a good stretch. Now return to the upright position and bend your knees to pick up your walking stick before the light changes. If you have an audience by now, bow and smile!

Near the completion of your walk (2 to 3 blocks from your destination) you can work on improving your coordination. Hold the stick off the ground about 12 inches in front of you near the center of your body and kick it gently, first with one foot and then the other. The object is to see how many times you can kick the stick without missing. You will be surprised to discover within a short period of time how easily you are able to kick the stick for blocks without missing a beat.

Another use that can be made of the walking stick is to help you become more proficient in a sports activity. Again, while waiting for the light to change, you can practice your golf swing . . . or imagine yourself as Billie Jean King making contact with a tennis ball . . . or a baton twirler leading the Rose Bowl Parade . . . or a fencer. The number of activities you can practice is unlimited. Rehearsing different aspects of your favorite sport while walking can produce significant improvement. All you need besides your walking stick is a little imagination.

There is no need to go out and purchase an expensive walking stick. Pick up a dead tree limb, whittle it down, and shape it to your specification. Then put it near the door so you won't forget to take it with you on your early morning and late evening walks. It can become a pleasurable companion and, in a matter of weeks, an aid that you will not want to be without.

Pedometer

A pedometer is a small precision instrument that can be hooked to your belt, trousers, or skirt. It has a stride setting mechanism on the side that can be adjusted to your personal stride length and an internal pendulum that registers each stride to record the number of miles walked. There are several types of pedometers on the market, but the one that I am most familiar with is round and will probably remind you of a stop watch or pocket watch. The number of miles walked is recorded (up to 25) inside the facing and there is a resetting mechanism on the back. The accumulated miles are not easily erased accidentally on this type of pedometer, as is true of some. (Being able to preserve the number of miles walked has distinct advantages, as I will explain momentarily.) I do not wish to name a particular brand but I do recommend the type just described because it has proven to be the most durable and dependable for the people in my walking programs. Pedometers can be purchased from most sporting goods stores, and operational instructions are provided. If you have trouble finding a pedometer of the type I have recommended, ask the clerk in your local sporting goods store if you might look through some of the store's catalogues and order one, either through the store or directly through the mail.

If you are prone to fatigue while walking and do not want to walk more than your condition dictates, or if you are walking in an unfamiliar area without street signs or markers to indicate how far you have traveled, a pedometer is an essential aid. But as a way to monitor your daily walking progress and as a motivator to keep you walking, a pedometer is invaluable. Once you have set a daily walking goal, you are able to see at a quick glance, any time during the day, the number of miles you have walked. Since your pedometer is designed to give you immediate feedback, your level of awareness about walking is likely to remain quite high. Thus you can quickly determine the number of miles needed to achieve your daily goal and gauge your walking for the remainder of the day accordingly.

Since the pedometer I recommend can record the number of miles walked up to 25, many walkers prefer not to reset it at the end of a walk, but rather, to see how many days it takes to walk 25 miles. Others prefer to reset their pedometers each night and note the number of miles walked each day on their calendars. Thus the approach to using the pedometer as an aid is an individual one, so I urge you to try both approaches on alternate weeks and then decide which works best for you. The idea is simply to find ways in which you can use the pedometer to maintain and increase your motivation for walking, while having fun at the same time.

Although the pedometer has the capacity to give you immediate feedback on the number of miles walked, it cannot tell you how fast you are walking. Is that an issue for you at this point? No problem! With your pedometer at-

tached to your belt and a wrist watch you can easily determine the rate of speed at which you are walking. If you
walked 1 mile in 20 minutes, you were walking at the rate
of 3 miles per hour; if you walked 1 mile in 15 minutes, you
were walking 4 miles per hour; and so on.

Within several months, you can stop wearing a watch, if
you wish, and use your pedometer as a timepiece. Once you
are aware of your walking speed, you can look at the clock
before you leave the house, compute the minutes it will take
you to get where you are going at X miles per hour, and take
off walking. I do it all the time. I know how fast I walk and
how far I have to walk, so when I have my pedometer on
(which is just about always), I don't need a watch. I have to
brag a little bit and tell you that I am almost never late for
an appointment.

Let me take a minute here to tell you why I am sometimes
without a pedometer. I have a tendency to give mine away.
When my program participants say they are not wearing
theirs because they are broken, I lend them mine. If I am
asked about mine by a stranger on the street who seems, as
we talk, to have the potential to become a serious walker, I
am apt as not to give the stranger mine as an incentive. Of
course I keep a good supply in my office and at home, so I
am usually only a few hours away from having one again,
but I feel a little uneasy until I have replaced it.

I put on my pedometer as automatically as most people
reach for their watches, wallets, and keys. Since I don't own
a car, and very seldom have need for public transportation,
I am not uncomfortable leaving home without my wallet
and keys, but I really do not like being without my pedometer!

Going Public

While I am very high on the pedometer as a motivational
aid, I do not want to lead you down the primrose path and
delude you into believing that simply wearing a pedometer

is a panacea for a walker. As with many aids, strategies, and activities, the enthusiasm for using a pedometer is sometimes short-lived, but this need not be the case. One way to prevent this from happening (and I am sure you can think of others) is to "Go Public." Let me explain it this way: With the purchase of this book, you have made a private commitment to walking. With the purchase of a pedometer, you will have made still another private commitment to walking. But in order to receive the full reinforcing benefits, your pedometer should be displayed publicly. You should wear it hanging outside your skirt or trousers in public view. You want the world to know that you are a walker who walks X number of miles a day or a week and that you have an instrument to prove it. In time, you will become somewhat of a celebrity in your office or neighborhood, but you must be ready to pay the price for this new status. For example, people who see you every day will begin to stop you to see if you are maintaining the walking level that you set last week. Some will ask "Is that all you have walked today?" It will soon become apparent to your friends and family that you are a serious walker.

Others will begin asking you about how the pedometer works. Great! Take that opportunity to begin proselytizing. Get on your soapbox and talk about the walking experience. Explain how the pedometer is helping to keep your motivation up and is making walking a more exciting venture.

Once you go public, turning back will be difficult because others will begin to have certain expectations of you. The expectations of others, however, will not present a problem if you are consistent and have a realistic walking goal that you can attain every day or every week.

A word on care and maintenance. Most pedometers are damaged when they are dropped or slip off the belt or trousers and fall on the floor or street. During the first couple of days of wearing yours, check occasionally to see if it is fitting snugly. If you are in the habit of letting your skirt or trousers hit the floor when you take them off, try to remember your reliable and dependable friend and motivator. The type of work you do is also a factor since bending and rubbing up against objects in the area where your pedometer is attached may affect its stability. With proper care and attention, your pedometer will last for years.

A word of caution, though. Spouses, children, and friends are often fascinated by a pedometer and will ask to wear it. There is a high probability that a borrowed pedometer will be returned broken. Consequently, you should be careful about lending it, because you might be without your valuable aid for days or weeks and this could adversely affect your adherence to your walking schedule.

Walking Chart

The walking chart is another valuable walking aid. It is easy to construct, it costs practically nothing, and it is simple to use. By placing your walking chart in a conspicuous spot in your home or office you will have a visible reminder that will increase your awareness of your commitment to walking. You will be setting up a competition—with yourself.

A walking chart is a way of illustrating graphically the number of miles you walk over several days or weeks and is very useful in maintaining or increasing your motivation to achieve a short-range or long-range walking goal. Finally, the chart can serve as a permanent record that will allow you to analyze your own walking progress over time.

While the walking stick and pedometer are aids that require a minimal amount of time and effort on your part, I must warn you that a walking chart will require a few minutes of your time each day. Are the benefits worth it? Obviously, I think so. But the only way you can determine just how valuable it is is to try it out for several weeks. Experiment with as many aids as you can, including a walking chart, and then decide which aid or combination of aids is enjoyable, is able to motivate you to continue walking, and is compatible with your daily routine.

Assignment: Construct a Walking Chart

You do not have to be a draftsman to construct a walking chart, but you will need a pencil, a ruler (or other straight-edge), and a blank piece of paper about the size of notebook or typing paper. I have illustrated a walking chart on the next page for you to use as your guide. As you can see, the chart I drew is for someone who might expect to walk 1 to 7 miles per day and the period of time I have reflected is a week in August. This hypothetical walker walked 4 miles on the 8th, 5 miles on the 9th, 3 miles on the 10th, and so forth.

TIME OUT FOR ME
WHILE YOU DRAW YOUR CHART

SAMPLE WALKING CHART

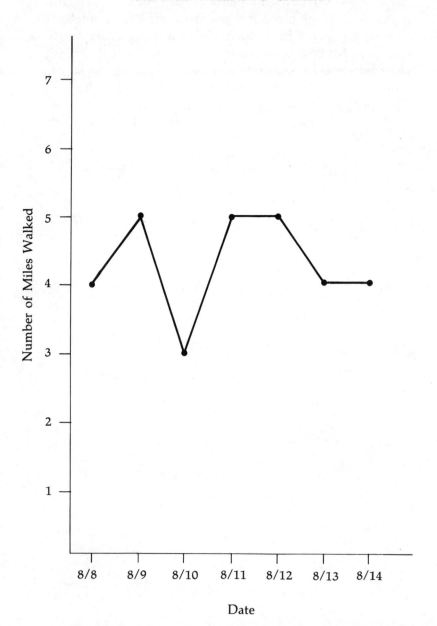

Did you draw a weekly chart? A two-week one? The whole month? Before you actually begin recording anything on it, you might consider covering up the specific dates and duplicating the form if you have access to a machine. Perhaps you could walk to the closest fast-copy center right now and have a supply of forms made for the coming weeks?

Whether you duplicate your chart on a copier or draw a new one for each new time period, you might want to think of ways to make it especially attractive. Be creative! Draw some flowers around the border, cut out a picture of a person walking and paste it at the top, or use more than one color of pencil or pen to make it more colorful. The idea is to construct a chart that reflects the new you!

Charlene, a participant in one of my weight management groups, worked as a sales representative. She did not embellish her walking chart or put it on the front of her refrigerator as I often suggest. She did, however, find a conspicuous place in her office, next to her sales chart. (As an incentive to increase sales, many companies give monthly awards or annual profit shares, so she had for many years kept a sales chart behind her desk to graph her monthly record.) Charlene even added a third chart, one on which she could record her weight loss. She wanted to be able, for the duration of the weight management program, to tell at a glance exactly what kind of progress she was making. Eureka! It worked! Within a matter of weeks, she became an office celebrity.

As might be expected, fellow employees focused on her consistent 1 to 2 pound a week weight loss and ignored the walking chart. It didn't take long for a consistent and serious walker to alter that, though, as she began sharing with her fellow workers how walking was changing her body and her life. Fellow workers started coming by for consultation: Where do I purchase a pedometer? How far should I walk? When and where should I walk? Where can I purchase a pair of walking shoes? And instead of checking her pedometer, they stopped by to check her walking chart for consistency.

(Of course, competing sales representatives also took a quick peek at her sales chart.)

Did walking increase her sales? I cannot say the extent, if at all, to which her walking influenced her monthly sales, but her upward spiral did continue. I can also tell you that she generated a lot of enthusiasm in her office, that she apparently helped keep up her own motivation for walking by helping others, and that before she finished the weight management program she was within 10 pounds of her ideal weight. Sales, weight loss, and walking . . . Ah, the sweet smell of success!

Analyzing Your Walking Habits

Many times over the course of several weeks you may not be able to identify the reason why you walked less or more on certain days, but by examining your walking chart—that permanent and reliable record—you may be able to recall specific factors that interfered or that prevented you from walking more. Conversely, the chart may help you recall why certain days were more productive in terms of walking. This is what I was alluding to when I mentioned using a walking chart to analyze your walking behavior.

For instance, by reviewing your walking chart for the past 2 weeks, you may discover that when you did not reach your walking goal on certain days it was because of inclement weather, house guests, a family emergency, an injury, a vacation or business trip, or ferocious neighborhood dogs. My response to all of these excuses, which you are offering as "legitimate reasons," is that you are selling yourself a bill of goods. It's a cop-out! It just may well be that you need to review the chapters on when and where to walk, or your walking schedule. Did you forget about Alice and how she handled house guests? You can do it too, but you will have to start getting tough with yourself, and with your friends, family, and co-workers as well.

I am not referring to physical toughness where you walk despite the pain, but mental toughness where you continue to say to yourself, "I can and I will go for a _____ mile walk _____ days this week." The message is clear. When it appears that external events are interfering with your walking, review your walking chart and get tough, mentally.

There are additional ways to use your walking chart for self-analysis of your walking behavior. How about a return to the basics? If the words GRADUALISM, CONSISTENCY, and ENJOYMENT immediately come to mind, we are in sync. While you cannot determine, based on your walking chart, whether you had fun or not (unless you made a special notation), the high points on your walking chart may act as a stimulus for recalling some enjoyable moments on those days. Your walking chart will also provide extremely important information on the other two basic elements, gradualism and consistency.

In reviewing your walking chart, ask yourself the following questions: Does my chart reflect a gradual increase based on my physical condition? Am I a consistent walker? Am I consistently inconsistent? A cursory examination of this valuable aid will answer all of the questions immediately. Your inconsistency will stand out like a sore thumb since the number of miles walked will be down in black and white.

A zigzag pattern or a lot of peaks and valleys on your walking chart will reflect inconsistency only if it is unintentional. If you have worked out a walking program in which you are using a hard-easy approach on alternate days, you are, in fact, doing what I recommend. Even so, there should not be more than a 50% deviation from one day to the next. In other words, if you are walking 8 miles on your hard day, you should be walking at least 4 miles on your easy day.

In sum, don't get into the habit of inserting the number of miles walked day after day without analyzing your walking behavior. Review your chart periodically. Look at how far you have come and give yourself a pat on the back!

Walking across America

While a walking chart can be used as a motivator for an individual or a group and is often more advantageous than a pedometer, a map of your city, state, or the United States is often even more beneficial. By adding a $1.25 map to your armamentarium of aids, you can bring a new dimension to your ever-expanding walking experience. Simply put, I am talking about an imaginary walk across America. I am talking about letting your fantasies go and basking in the beauty of sections of this country that you may never visit in person. In essence, I am talking about patriotism. Yes, I know I have said it before, and I am saying it here, and I will say it again before I complete this book: WALKING IS . . . PATRIOTIC.

An imaginary walk across America is even more than a patriotic act. It's a low-cost vacation, a new and exciting way to see the United States, a lesson in history, a family project, a group reinforcer. More important still, it is a way to keep you walking for years without getting bored.

This is an ambitious undertaking that will require considerable time and effort on your part. It will necessitate attention to a host of details as well as the dogged determination to go it alone, if necessary, to achieve a long-range walking goal. How does it work? Let's use as an example a map of the United States.

Suppose you would set an individual goal of walking from New York City to Los Angeles. Next suppose you select 20 places of interest (say every 500 miles) that you would like to visit along your walking route. There are no time constraints involved, so all you need to do is purchase a map, set a reasonable walking goal (daily, weekly, monthly), and take off walking on your imaginary trip. As always, your primary goal is to have fun every step of the way.

Each week or each month, total up the number of miles walked and graph them on your map as you would with a walking chart. Most maps include a scale of inches to miles that you can use to measure the distance between your chosen points of interest. For example, if 1 inch equals 100 miles on your map, you will probably want to accumulate your walking mileage in 25-mile blocks and then plot your progress ¼ inch from your starting place. If you anticipate feeling discouraged at the prospects of moving at this pace, you can move across the map faster by deciding that you will credit yourself with 10 miles on the map for every 1 mile actually walked. Using this formula, you would be able to cover 1 inch, or 100 miles, with each 10 miles walked.

Now comes the fantasy and fun part. Several weeks before you reach one of the places that you plan to visit, go to the library and check out several books on the area. Better yet, if you have your course laid out, write the Chamber of Commerce of the city or the Tourist Bureau for that state and tell them you plan to be in that area in a few weeks and would like maps, pamphlets, and other literature on places of interest. Begin reading about different sights and making plans to visit them when you arrive. Once you reach the first place of interest and take several imaginary walks and go sightseeing, begin making plans for the next place of interest about 500 miles away.

Am I making you weary before you begin your imaginary walk? Is the immensity of the task overwhelming? If the basic idea appeals to you, don't give it up. Get tough mentally. Why not turn this novel idea into a group project and enlist the help of your family? You have virtually nothing to lose and you stand to gain more than you might expect. For instance, it may have an educational impact on your children and grandchildren. Since history is often a fairly boring subject, a walk across America with your family just may make history come alive. With Dad, who has always been lukewarm to visiting certain sites on vacation, an imaginary walk across America might be the spark that will light a fire under him. Once you get him emotionally involved in the project and physically committed to it, there is a 50-50

chance that he will change his mind about some of his vacation ideas. The old saying, "It's not what you do, but how
you do it" is another way of saying that you should be
diplomatic in your introduction of this idea to your family.
Show your optimism without being overbearing, and let
your commitment to the idea speak for itself. Walk! At best,
you will be well-informed about America to the point that
when questions arise about history, geography, regional culture, or a dream place for a vacation, you will have a ready
response.

OK, so the family is resistant to the notion. Your father
is playing golf, your mother just joined the local spa and
paid for a lifetime membership, your husband is playing
tennis four times a week—or your wife is jogging. Your
children and grandchildren are also too busy rollerskating,
skateboarding, and playing racquetball. Are you ready to
throw in the towel and say it will not work? But it will work!
How about sharing this idea with some of your friends in
the neighborhood or at church? If all else fails, start your
own walking group and let the group decide whether a city,
state, regional, or United States map is best. You do not have
to walk together every day as a group. Just have each group
member report the number of miles walked each week or
month, sum up the miles walked, and draw a line on your
map. Give the group feedback on their progress and encourage them to continue walking.

Since most of my weight management groups are limited
to 12 or 24 weeks, I use a regional map and try to encourage
the groups to set realistic goals. When we total up the miles
once a week and draw a line on the map I realize how much
enthusiasm the map generates in the group. The beauty of
it is that it is also non-competitive. Group members are not
competing with each other but are making a contribution to
a group goal that is based on each member's personal walking goal. As the instigator of your own group project you
will not have to exert pressure on yourself to make a valuable contribution—the enthusiasm of the group will do that

and you will find that you are walking more and more miles each week.

Whether you take your imaginary walks alone or as part of a group effort, remember that the journey is the key to enjoyment—not the destination itself. So lay your course out across America and walk. When you arrive at one of the sights you have selected, close your eyes and think about all the wonderful things you read about the waterfall, the snow-capped mountains in July, the barren desert, and so forth. Your feet will get you there, and your imagination will take care of the rest.

Choosing Your Own Aids

Assuming that you either already had good walking shoes or have now purchased a pair, I want you to choose two of the other aids (walking stick, pedometer, walking chart, or map) that you can incorporate into your daily routine as motivators. Based on my experience with a number of successful and not-so-successful walkers, you stand a 60% chance of becoming addicted to walking if you use two out of the four aids consistently. The odds increase in your favor as you increase your use of aids. Selecting three out of four aids will increase your chance of success to 80%, and using all four will assure you a 90% chance. There is no 100% guarantee; however, you can stack the deck in your favor by using these aids—or by using your own imagination to develop other more suitable ones for your particular situation.

7

Getting the Most Out of Each Step

Now that you are moving along at a comfortable pace with your two walking aids, you are ready to shift your attention to some additional factors associated with the walking experience: your attitude, breathing, posture, walking style, and the care of the most maligned part of your body, your feet. Each of these factors, if approached individually, will yield additional benefits. To intensify those benefits, though, and to expand the walking experience to another level and get the most out of each step, you must practice putting all of these factors together in a gradual and consistent manner.

Mental Attitude

A positive mental attitude is the first factor that you must concentrate on and practice to get the most out of each step. Your attitude reflects how you feel about yourself and the world around you, and in many respects, it sets the tone for your day. Thus it is crucial that you get yourself in the right frame of mind and think positively, not only during your walk, and after your walk, but before your walk.

For me, it begins when I first awaken, yawn, and stretch. Often I repeat the popular expression, "Today is the first day of the rest of my life." On other occasions, I make up my own positive statements.

There are several important considerations to keep in

mind if you are going to construct your own positive state-ments. For one, each statement should include such verbs as *will, am, is, can.* Make sure that your statement is potent enough to have an impact that will last 16 to 18 hours. Quite simply, the goal, even before you get out of bed, is to give yourself a positive message that will stay with you through-out the day.

True, there will be days when personal concerns will over-whelm you, and I readily admit that sometimes the problems of the world are cause for a pessimistic attitude. The key question you must ask yourself when this occurs is: Will being gloomy and depressed about personal problems and bemoaning the sad state of the world (which, by the way, may not be quite as bad as it seems at times) solve the problem or change the world? Highly unlikely! You can, however, go for a walk and think through your personal problems or concerns. Furthermore, during your walk you may come up with some alternatives related to the world situation (or at least some local community problem) that you can share with public officials. Better yet, how about organizing in your head a letter to the editor of your local paper stating your position on inflation, foreign policy, crime, unemployment, and other issues? (You might even actually sit down and write it when you get home.) At any rate, adopting a positive attitude and going for a walk are steps in the right direction!

Whether you are going to be pessimistic or optimistic about your day is under your control, and since you are the master of your own thoughts, you definitely have a choice to make each day. If you think negative thoughts through-out the day, is it any wonder that nothing goes right? On the other hand, you can use a positive mental attitude and opti-mism as your guiding light whereby you tune in and become amenable to all of the positive things that are happening in your environment. The self-fulfilling prophecy that today is going to be a terrible day will become a reality if you con-tinue to accent and orient your thoughts in a negative direc-tion. It is important to remember that the power to change the situation has also been invested in you. You can turn defeat into victory, you can become an eternal optimist, and you can make today a good day, this week a good week, and this month and this year the best ever. The '80s can be the happiest decade you have known. But in order for this to happen, you must practice, starting today, the art of cultivating a positive mental attitude.

Do I hear you saying that you have heard this positive pitch before and that you are unimpressed? My response is that your skepticism is probably based on what happened yesterday. What I am talking about is today and all of your tomorrows. Therefore, I can only urge you to try again and to tell yourself before you start that this approach will work for you!

Are you with me? OK! Before you go to bed tonight, write a positive statement on a piece of paper, read it several times, and place it on your bedside table before you drift off to sleep. (The statement can be one you have heard or read or one of your own making.) When you awaken, read the statement several times or until you have committed it to memory. Look in a mirror after you get out of bed, smile, and repeat your positive statement. (One of my friends always laughs when she talks to herself in the mirror, but that, too, is a good way to start the day.) Later, as you walk out the door, continue smiling and repeating your statement. As you walk through your neighborhood, be pleasant. Smile. Don't be afraid to say, Hello . . . Good Morning . . . Good Afternoon . . . Good Evening. Say it with gusto! Your enthusiasm and optimism will be contagious and just might uplift the spirit of others. But more important, you will have brightened your own day.

Breathing

The second factor associated with getting the most out of each step is an activity that is as natural to man as walking: breathing. At rest, approximately 5 liters of air are inhaled by the lungs every minute; however, the lungs have the capacity to inhale 100 liters per minute while you are engaging in strenuous muscular activity such as brisk walking.

You need not wait until you go for a walk to begin to increase the capacity of your lungs. You can practice inhaling deeply and exhaling slowly while you are sitting in your comfortable chair reading this book, or while standing at the counter of a store waiting to be checked out. Let me briefly explain the inhalation-exhalation process.

During inhalation, air enters through the nostrils, and the diaphragm descends. This pushes the abdomen out slightly, causing negative pressure in the chest. This, in turn, causes the lungs to expand and draw in air. The surface of the lungs is covered with millions of tiny air sacs, called alveoli, which transfer oxygen into your red blood corpuscles. This oxygen is then carried throughout your body to nourish every cell.

Exhalation is a passive process, but one that is extremely important in the completion of the breathing cycle. Exhalation involves a relaxation of the respiratory muscle, a gradual pulling in of the stomach, and an emptying of the lungs in preparation for the next breath. During exhalation, the air sacs lining the lungs take the waste (carbon dioxide) from the red corpuscles, and this waste is then expelled to the outer atmosphere with each breath.

One way to conceptualize the breathing process is to think of your lungs as a deflated balloon. With the inhalation of air, imagine that you are blowing up the balloon. As all parts of the lungs are filled, feel the fullness in your chest and lower back. Then, as you exhale, imagine that you are slowly letting the air out of the balloon and concentrate on the feeling of flatness in your chest and stomach.

The recommended inhalation-exhalation ratio is 1:2. In other words, exhalation should take twice as long as inhalation. In both instances, however, the process should be effortless, and should occur naturally and rhythmically. Are you ready for a practice session? Good!

First, sit in a straight-backed chair with your body reflecting good posture. Breathe normally for a few minutes. Now breathe in deeply through your nostrils in a relaxed manner and count to 2 (one thousand and one, one thousand and two). Now exhale through your mouth and count to 4 (one thousand and one, one thousand and two, one thousand and three, one thousand and four). Repeat this procedure twice. The third time, close your eyes and get a picture of a candle flickering in front of you. Now blow out the candle, not with one puff, but with a smooth, constant flow of air. Do you feel a little more relaxed? Have you reached your physical limit? If so, practice at the present level for several days.

Once you are comfortable inhaling for 2 seconds and exhaling for 4 seconds, try a 3-second (inhale) and 6-second (exhale) cycle, and then a 4- and 8-second cycle. Concentrate on inhaling through your nostrils until your lungs are filled to capacity, then slowly exhale until you feel that every ounce of air has been expelled. Then pull your stomach in a little more to force the last bit of air out of your lungs. When you have completed this exercise, repeat it standing up.

As you are walking, the same 1:2 ratio applies. Try to coordinate your breathing with each step. For instance, breathe in for 4 steps then breathe out for 8 steps. Keep an even, natural walking stride with your arms swinging gently. Let your breathing flow smoothly with the natural rhythm of your body. And don't forget to blow out the candle as you walk.

If you are just recovering from surgery, or have emphysema, or are severely overweight, this might be difficult at first. But whatever your current physical condition, your respiration will improve with practice. Follow the gradual and consistent approach that you are using to increase your walking. By all means, stay with whatever breathing ratio is most comfortable for you before moving to a longer inhalation-exhalation cycle.

Posture

Can you recall being told by one of your parents or your health education teachers to sit up straight in your seat, or to walk with your head erect, chest out, and stomach in? The reason you were admonished to sit and walk tall is because poor posture not only affects your appearance but is also a bad habit that is hard to correct. In addition, when your body is not properly aligned, you miss some very important benefits.

Slouch down in your chair and exhibit the worst possible sitting posture. Now inhale and exhale for 30 seconds. OK! Now sit up straight in your chair with your head erect, chest out, and stomach in and inhale and exhale for 30 seconds exhibiting good posture. Did you notice that it was more difficult to breathe when you were sitting with your body reflecting poor posture? Since you had to expend more energy forcing the air out of your lungs, your breathing was probably shallow. On the other hand, unless you have emphysema or some other health problem, breathing while sitting straight was almost effortless, and muscle expenditure was minimal. Thus good sitting, standing, and walking posture will facilitate breathing and will expand your lung capacity. In most instances, poor posture is just a bad habit that you have developed over the years, and you can change any habit with practice.

Since the benefits that you receive from correcting your sitting and standing posture will be socially and physically reinforcing, there is a good likelihood that you will want to improve your walking posture as well. This logical progression is not surprising inasmuch as improvement in one area will make you aware of the need for improvement in another area. Are you aware of how your body looks when you are walking? If not, you might want to take a few minutes to do the mirror test. The objectives of the test are to ascertain if your body is properly aligned while standing and walking. After you complete the mirror test, I will point out a few fun ways to assess and correct your posture on your next walk.

Without the aid of an expert, one way to have your posture assessed is to have a member of your family or a friend observe you walking and give you feedback on different aspects of your walking posture. But this is not always possible or necessary. A more practical "do it yourself" way is to observe your body as you walk toward a full-length mirror. Stand facing the mirror approximately 15 feet away and examine your body for a moment. Now with your natural style of walking, walk toward the mirror and stop after 5 steps. Repeat this procedure several times and systematically examine your body from your head to your feet each time you approach the mirror.

Do you see a need for improvement in any area? If not, fine! But let's say you notice that certain parts of your body are not properly aligned. For instance, your head is tilted to the left, your left shoulder is noticeably lower than the right one, and your right foot is slightly slewed. Unless you are overly compulsive about changing such postural defects and are willing to stand in front of a mirror practicing proper body alignment, you will probably forget about them after the test. A better way is to develop techniques in your natural walking environment that will be just as effective in assessing and correcting your walking posture as the ones mentioned above but that will also be fun.

Fun Ways to Assess Your Posture

While walking, focus on a tree or some other straight object several blocks away and align your body with that object. Walk toward that object as if you were going to walk through it, keeping your body as straight as possible. As you come within 25 or 30 feet of the object, select another object in the distance and repeat the same procedure. Although you might not be able to align your body entirely, this procedure will make you more aware of your posture as you are walking.

The sun and the moon are excellent guides for assessing and correcting postural defects. Unfortunately, 365 days of sunshine and a full moon every night are luxuries that we cannot always count on, but on those occasions when the sun is shining or the moon is glowing brightly behind you, your body will cast a shadow in front of you. It is time for shadow watching.

Look at your shadow to see if your head is tilted, shoulders slouched, arms swinging, and so forth. Then observe how your shadow makes the adjustment when you straighten your head and pull back your shoulders in an erect position. And then when you get around to taking one of those late-night strolls I mentioned earlier, holding hands in the moonlight with your favorite person, check out your shadow and adjust your body accordingly.

By now you may also have begun observing the postures you see in other walkers. If so, have any of those walkers influence you? In what ways? It may be helpful to use the perfect walking posture of another person as a model or as a way to get a mental image of how your body looks moving in space. Emulate those you meet who have beautiful carriage and soon you will be walking in a similar manner. People watching is an excellent way, without the aid of the sun, moon, a straight object, or a reflective device, to maintain a high level of awareness about your walking posture.

I must point out, though, that despite herculean efforts to change the way you walk, there are individual factors that influence your posture. For instance, have you gained a substantial amount of weight in the last 5 to 10 years? If so, this extra weight has probably caused you to walk differently in order to maintain your balance and to support the additional weight.

As you get older there is also a loss of neuromuscular functioning; therefore, to increase stability, you might have changed the angle of your foot several degrees. Then too, there are role models after whom you have patterned yourself. (Do you walk like your mother or father because you were born that way or because you observed them walking that way for many years?) Further, there are structural and congenital defects such as being slew-footed or knock-kneed to which your body has accommodated itself over the years.

No amount of practice will make you walk straight if you are extremely slew-footed. Surgery or braces may improve the situation, but practice will probably have little effect. In fact, to practice trying to turn your foot inward could be more damaging than if you just accept it as a slight variation in your otherwise-perfect walking style.

The point that I am making is that, while you may have some limitations, you can still enjoy the walking experience. Accept your limitations and continue walking. You do not want to become so preoccupied with assessing and correcting your posture that you miss the main point of this chapter —and of this book—body awareness and fun. The goal is to find the happy medium.

Walking Style

As I indicated earlier, there is a distinct relationship between your mental attitude, your breathing, and your walking posture. But the logical progression does not end there. These factors work together to form your own, very personal walking style. Your mental attitude affects your posture, your posture affects your breathing, and your mental attitude, posture, and breathing affect your walking style. Sometimes this scenario works in a negative direction. You go out for a walk, in a bad mood, and are probably slouching. As your breathing becomes laborious, your body gets heavy and tired after walking a few blocks, so you discontinue your walk and head for your easy chair, where you think more negative thoughts. This vicious cycle can be broken by answering one question: How do you look and act when you feel good about yourself? In all likelihood, your mood is lighter, you probably smile more, and enthusiasm shows on your face. The movement of your body is quite different because you walk to the beat of your own drum with authority and confidence. And guess what! When you walk this way you are putting all the factors together naturally. That, fellow walkers, is the essence of an efficient walking style that is exclusively yours. You felt that way and walked tall to the beat of your own drum yesterday or last week. Can you walk that way every day? Why not?

Are you walking tall? Is your head erect? Shoulders back? Chest high? Stomach pulled in? Knees and feet pointed in the direction that you are walking? Begin thinking tall when you sit and stand, and each time you go for a walk, tell yourself that you are an inch taller than your last measured height. As you walk and practice extending your body slightly upward, you will, in fact, increase your height half an inch to an inch.

Are you walking to the beat of your own drum? That is, are you walking with an even, smooth-flowing walking style that is in concert with the natural rhythm of your body? Since you are not competing in a race, speed and stride are not important. Concentrate on finding the pace that is best for you. Easy does it as you let your body take over and do its own thing. Let your arms, which are bent slightly at the elbows, swing gently from the shoulders, in perfect rhythm with the movement of the opposite leg.

In sum, to get the most out of each step you must become more aware of your body as it moves in space, and practice, based on your physical limitations, in a gradual and consistent manner, putting all of the factors together. Before your next walk, get those positive thoughts flowing and smile as you prepare yourself for a total body approach to walking.

For the first 5 minutes, concentrate on your breathing. Inhale naturally and deeply and then exhale and push the air out of your lungs in a slow, relaxed manner. The second 5 minutes can be devoted to your walking posture. Concentrate on holding your head straight, keeping your shoulders erect and your chest high, and pulling in your stomach. Within a brief period of time, it will all fit together naturally.

As you continue to practice assessing and correcting specific features associated with your unique walking style, something extraordinary will happen from your head to your feet. You will discover that a pleasant thought can set the tone for your day and your walk. You will find that your rhythmic breathing facilitated by your erect posture will coalesce with your smooth, even-flowing, relaxed walking style. Further, you will experience the joyful, magical sensation that comes when your body takes over as you hit your natural stride, totally oblivious to your surroundings. Soon practicing will become a secondary issue because you will have searched and found the natural body rhythm that is perfect for you. And that walking nirvana, that euphoric state attained by serious and committed walkers, is one step away.

The Prime Movers: Your Feet

Are you one of the 189 million Americans who spend millions of dollars each year on their feet? I was, until I started giving my feet the attention they really deserve.

Since you were probably not born with bad feet but developed any problems you might have in this area early in life, there is a good chance that foot care and foot exercises will increase your walking pleasure. You do not have to resign yourself to aching feet and to purchasing over-the-counter foot products for the remainder of your life. In fact, if you have been reading this book carefully and doing the assignments, you have already taken steps to prevent a lot of common problems that occur from ill-fitting shoes, poor posture, and poor walking style. My objectives are straightforward: to elevate your awareness about an important but neglected area of your body; to point out ways to incorporate foot exercises into your normal daily routine; and to make the care of your feet a high-priority item.

The main purpose of the foot is to provide support, balance, and locomotion. In addition, the foot absorbs the impact of each step and is responsible for the distribution of the weight of the body. Thus determining whether your feet are pointed in the direction that you are walking and correcting the way your heel strikes the walking surface are obvious concerns. You do not want to look at your feet every step of your walk, so let me share a few quick ways to evaluate whether you are walking straight. Then I would like for you to be creative and think of some other ways of checking your progress.

Of course, you can retake the mirror test and focus specifically on your feet as you approach the mirror. Or, after you take a bath or shower, walk on a hardwood floor or linoleum before drying your feet. If you live near a beach, check out your footprints in the sand. Simple assessment procedures like these will give you a general idea of how your heel strikes the walking surface and whether you are pushing off on the ball of your foot or on the outer edge of your foot. You can also evaluate your heel strike and "toe-off" by simply looking at several pairs of your old shoes. A heel that is worn down near the center and a bald spot in the region of the ball of your foot suggest that your heel strike is adequate and that you are pushing off with your toes correctly. If, on the other hand, the outer edge of the heel and the outer edge near the little toe are worn down heavily in a lopsided manner, your heel strike is causing your fourth and fifth toes to bear too much of the responsibility for propulsion. This type of toe-off leads to poor support and balance, a reduction in speed, and increased injuries.

If you are having difficulty in walking straight, draw two imaginary lines, 6 inches apart, 50 to 75 feet in front of you. Now walk on them. Or you may prefer to focus on one foot at a time. If so, the next time you are walking on a tiled surface, or any other surface with intersecting lines, try placing your heel down on the middle of the line and having the line come between the first and second toe. In this position, the foot is facing straight ahead, the knee is in a direct line with the foot, and the hip is in a position to receive maximal rotation for its range of motion. Walk for several blocks with your right foot walking the line, then walk with the left foot on the line for several blocks. Finally, center your body over the line and walk placing each foot down pointing straight ahead.

Lifetime Wear and Tear

To illustrate the amount of impact that your foot sustains throughout your life, a simple computation will make the point. For the purpose of this illustration, I will use a life expectancy of 70 years and an estimate that the average person will walk 2 miles per day throughout a lifetime.

$$\begin{array}{rl} 365 & \text{days per year} \\ \times\ \ \ 2 & \text{miles per day} \\ \hline 730 & \text{miles per year} \end{array} \quad\text{and}\quad \begin{array}{rl} 730 & \text{mile per year} \\ \times\ \ 70 & \text{years of age} \\ \hline 51{,}100 & \text{miles per lifetime} \end{array}$$

Thus a 70-year-old person who walks an average of 2 miles per day walks 51,100 miles in a lifetime. Let me translate that into steps.

One mile is equal to 5,280 feet and the average person's stride is 2 feet, so to find the number of steps taken per mile I can simply divide 5,280 by 2.

$$2\overline{)5280} \qquad 2640 \text{ steps per mile}$$

If you are interested in the number of steps the average person might take in a day, a year, or so forth, you can do your own computations.

$$\begin{array}{rl} 2640 & \text{steps per mile} \\ \times\ \ \ 2 & \text{miles per day} \\ \hline & \text{miles per day} \end{array} \quad\text{or}\quad \begin{array}{rl} 2640 & \text{steps per mile} \\ \times\ 730 & \text{miles per year} \\ \hline & \text{steps per year} \end{array}$$

$$\text{or}\quad \begin{array}{rl} 2640 & \text{steps per mile} \\ \times\ 51{,}100 & \text{miles per lifetime} \\ \hline & \text{steps per lifetime} \end{array}$$

Of course, you can personalize this procedure by inserting your age and the number of miles you are presently walking, which I assume is greater than the 2-mile number used here.

With each step, you exert 1 to 1½ times your body weight on each foot, so to determine the exact number of pounds of impact that you exert each day, year, or throughout your lifetime on your feet, multiply your weight by the number of steps you take for each of these time periods. As you will see, the figure may come to hundreds of tons.

Are you having fun with the numbers? If so, keep the game going. One way to have fun (and possibly to learn something new as well) is to go metric. Since going metric is a new American trend, how about computing kilograms of impact instead of pounds, and kilometers walking instead of miles? I think you've got the message.

Although no other part of your body could withstand being the main cushion for this constant impact, your feet continue to perform in spite of your inattention to them. For instance, you might think nothing of spending an hour a week at the barber shop or beauty salon, or 30 minutes on a home shampoo, a bedtime facial, or a daily bath, and another 30 minutes putting on makeup or shaving, combing your hair, and brushing your teeth. All of these activities are designed to make you look, smell, and feel better, but when you get out of the bathtub or shower, you probably blot your feet dry in 15 seconds and rush to dress. Unfair! Since your feet rank as among the most used parts of the body, they definitely deserve more attention and care.

Your feet also reflect the health of the body and are often used to diagnose many medical problems such as diabetes, arthritis, kidney disorders, and circulatory problems—so take a minute to examine your own feet. No, not tomorrow. Right now! (unless personal discretion indicates otherwise). Take off your shoes and your socks or hose, and examine your feet thoroughly. Look at the top of each foot, and between and under your toes. Inspect the heels, the balls of your feet, and your insteps. Examine all areas for discoloration, for dryness of skin, for brittle nails, for corns, bunions, warts, or blisters. Many of these conditions are early warning signs of systemic problems, especially in the elderly. If you see such warning signals, call your doctor.

Take Five

Your feet get just as tired as other parts of your body, so I recommend that you set aside at least 5 minutes each day for foot care. The following plan is designed to promote circulation in the lower extremities, to alleviate pain, to aid in the prevention of injuries, and to bring pleasure to your entire body.

The elevation of your feet, washing them, and massaging them are all important. While bathing or relaxing, and especially after walking, elevate your feet and let the blood drain back toward your heart. Flex your toes backward and forward while your feet are elevated and try to stretch your toes as far as possible for 3 to 5 seconds, then relax them. Repeat this procedure several times.

Your feet should be washed at least once a day with mild soap. Suds them thoroughly on the top, bottom, and between the toes. Rinse them thoroughly and pat them dry. Take a few extra seconds to dry between each toe, and apply a light coat of foot powder. The water softens the toenails, making them less brittle, so this is a good time to cut your toenails. As you well know, this is not necessary every day, but at least once every 2 weeks, trim your toenails straight across (that is, do not follow the curvature of the toes) to prevent ingrown toenails.

Massaging of the feet once they are dry should also occur every day. Pleasure your body by gently rubbing the top of each foot with your fingers and the palm of your hand, in an oval motion. With the palm of your hand, massage the heel and let your fingers move down the ball of the foot and massage this area. Next, gently massage the top, bottom, and between each toe. For a more soothing effect, use lotion or foot balm. Now grab the toes with one hand and the heel with the other and gently rotate your foot 5 times to the left and 5 times to the right. Do this to each foot. OK, your 5 minutes are up!

One way to get a natural massage is to walk barefooted. This allows for freedom of movement, the weight and balance of the body are distributed more evenly, and the feet are grounded in their natural state. Walking on sand, grass, or carpet helps to stimulate circulation, and bare feet receive ventilation after hours of being cooped up inside a shoe.

Daily Foot Exercises

There are a number of exercises that you can incorporate into your daily routine to strengthen your feet, ankles, and lower leg muscles to prevent injuries. I will mention a few that are part of my daily routine that you might modify to suit your particular situation. Be creative!

- After you complete your foot massage, or at other times when you are barefooted, try to pick up a marble or a pencil with your toes.
- Spread your toes as far apart as possible and hold for 5 seconds.
- With your shoes on, pull your toes up to the top of your shoes, then push them down, pressing your feet flat on the floor.
- Walk on the sides of your feet, 10 steps forward and 10 steps backward, once on the outer sides of your feet and once on the inner sides.
- While sitting, slowly raise your heel off the floor and simultaneously press the ball of your foot down, keeping your toes on the floor. Now let your heel return slowly to the floor. This is a good exercise for the calf.

- For a good achilles stretch, stand with your toes on top of a book that is 1 to 2 inches thick, raise your heels off the floor, and slowly return your heels to the floor. Do this several times, holding the stretch.
- Rotate your ankles throughout the day, and while you have them resting on an ottoman reading the evening newspaper, make it a habit to rotate them some more.

The message: Don't just sit or stand. Do something! Tighten and relax the muscles in your lower and upper leg, stretch your toes, rotate your feet. When and where? Anytime. Anywhere. When you are in a boring meeting, watching television, talking on the telephone, preparing dinner, or on one of those rare occasions (which I hope are becoming more and more infrequent) when you are riding in an automobile. Join me in adopting a new philosophy: I will not let my body remain motionless just because I am sitting or standing.

IMPORTANT POINTS TO REMEMBER

- A proper mental attitude is the first step to getting the most out of walking.
- Eternal optimists are made, not born.
- Proper breathing techniques and brisk walking will increase the capacity of the lungs to take in more air and remove waste from the body.
- A good inhalation-exhalation ratio is 1:2 and should be done naturally, slowly, deeply, and rhythmically.
- Good posture facilitates breathing.
- Poor posture throws the body out of line, and misalignment in one area causes misalignment in another area.
- A human carriage in motion is a thing of beauty.
- Shadow watching and using objects at a distance as a guide can improve your walking posture.
- Think tall, and you will walk tall.

- Walking a line with first one foot and then the other raises your level of awareness and improves your walking style.
- Proper care of the prime movers will increase your walking pleasure.
- Sing, hum, whistle, or smile as you walk and you will be the envy of your neighborhood.

8

Is That All There Is?

At this point you may be wondering if there is anything other than pleasure that you can gain from walking. There are other benefits and I have a hunch about them: Even by putting fun first as you are presently doing, you have probably already gained some of the additional benefits that I am about to describe.

Psychological Benefits

Since World War II, psychologists, psychiatrists, psychopharmacologists, physicians, and others have developed a number of techniques, devices, and pills for the purpose of treating anxiety, depression, and a host of other psychological problems. You have heard or read about most of them by now. Books, magazines, newspapers, and television advertisements continually recommend stimulants to get you going in the morning—and then routines that will help you relax at midmorning or evening—and finally, pills to help you sleep again at night. More and more frequently, though, members of the helping professions are recommending walking as a natural tension reducer and as one of the most effective ways of gaining inner peace.

The next time you are feeling overwhelmed by a personal problem, become self-reliant and go for a walk. You can do it immediately. There is no need to wait 4 or 8 hours to use this prescription. Even more important, it is available 24 hours a day and can be self-prescribed and self-administered anytime, at whatever dosage level fits your need!

Walking

- increases confidence
- reduces tension
- aids in problem solving
- provides a forum for relaxation and unwinding
- promotes a sense of general well-being
- is a positive way to handle anger
- is a pleasant distraction
- increases ability to handle stress
- adds life to your years
- helps to develop a positive body image
- stimulates the imagination
- reduces lethargy
- improves your disposition
- is a way to gain inner peace
- is noncompetitive
- improves your posture
- helps you to become mentally alert
- makes you self-reliant
- unclogs the mind
- helps you maintain mental equilibrium
- aids in developing a sense of humor
- brings creative impulses to the surface
- builds an appreciation of solitude
- is a way to reduce boredom
- sets the stage for meditation

Financial Benefits

Are there financial benefits associated with walking? This dollar and sense question is very timely since spending more and saving less is becoming a way of life for all too many

Americans. But this need not be the case. Would you believe I save $3500 a year by being an avid walker?

Three years ago I sold my car and became a foot traveler. Car payments, insurance premiums, gasoline, repair and maintenance costs, and parking fees are now a thing of the past—and I save in other ways as well. By walking downtown to make my monthly charge account payments and pay utility bills, I save on bus fare and postage (stamps will soon cost 25¢ each I am told!). I still go to my physician for an annual checkup, but I have not purchased any medication since I started walking. And just think of the money I've saved on speeding tickets. I have yet to hear of a person being ticketed for walking too fast!

I cannot in good conscience claim the entire $3500 figure as extra money in my pocket because I have one major expenditure that offsets a portion of this annual savings. Since I have become a serious and committed walker, I find that I need to buy a pair of good walking shoes about once a month, but that $400 a year is nothing compared to what most non-walkers spend on local transportation. I hope you will give serious consideration to walking as a way of saving money in the current inflationary period.

Walking

- is free
- saves you money at the gas station and in car repairs and maintenance
- cuts down on the need for prescribed drugs
- effects savings in doctor bills and hospitalization costs
- provides an opportunity for free family outings
- does not necessarily require special equipment
- increases work productivity
- aids in resiliency and recovery from injuries
- results in increased fitness and well-being at little cost
- results in the savings of dollars by not having to join a formal exercise or weight control program

- serves as an informal but highly visible neighborhood patrol that may reduce crime
- puts parking fee money back in your pocket
- is a good substitute for coffee and donuts during work breaks
- is a good substitute for lunch
- reduces hunger pangs
- is basically injury free
- facilitates weight loss and maintenance, thus eliminating the need to buy a new wardrobe in a larger size

According to Ray, a fellow walker, you do not necessarily have to increase the number of miles you walk each day or sell your car in order to receive the benefits outlined above. Three times a week, he walks 5 miles to his downtown law office, reviewing his cases and rehearsing his opening and closing arguments as he goes. Ray saves money on gas, parking, and bus fare and reports that his walking days seem to be his most creative and productive ones. Although these characteristics do not guarantee his winning every case, they surely do not contribute to his losses—and winning cases increases demand for his services. Thus walking not only saves money for Ray but may just possibly make money for him.

Physical Benefits

Are you able to play games with your children or grandchildren without getting exhausted? Can you climb several flights of stairs, carrying on a normal conversation, without using the bannister? If the answer to either one of the above questions is yes, then you have received some of the initial physical benefits associated with walking. As you continue walking, you will notice that the ordinary demands of daily life require less effort since your stamina, endurance, and energy level will have increased. Then, too, once you begin walking briskly, as many of you are doing already, the efficiency of your heart and lungs will increase. A quickened pace elevates your heart rate, and when your heart rate is elevated and sustained at a certain level, the muscles of the heart become stronger and the supply of oxygen throughout your body is increased. Thus to get to the heart of the matter and receive specific health benefits, you must step lively.

Brisk Walking

- increases cardiac output
- decreases blood pressure
- aids in sounder sleep
- increases respiration
- tones muscles
- increases collateral circulation
- increases blood supply to capillaries
- retards demineralization of bones
- aids in the maximal functioning of the skeletal system
- helps produce osteoblast bone cells
- reduces resting heart rate
- aids in weight loss and maintenance
- decreases appetite
- increases energy reserves
- improves balance and agility
- improves circulation
- is recommended for recuperation after surgery
- increases resiliency in case of injury
- improves skin tone
- aids in digestion and elimination
- aids in removal of fatty deposits from your arteries
- increases elasticity of arteries
- is good preventive medicine
- replaces fat with muscle
- promotes physical and mental health
- can save 10,000 to 20,000 heart beats each day
- strengthens the heart muscle
- decreases degenerative disease possibilities

Walking briskly is one way to "overload" or make an additional demand on your body to sustain an elevated heart rate. Increasing the distance walked or combining speed and distance are other ways. The objective, irrespective of the procedure you use to elevate your heart rate, is the same: to increase the circulation of your blood and the amount of oxygen you take into your lungs. Even though it is necessary to demand more of your body to receive physical benefits, you do not want to make drastic changes in your walking routine or to overexert yourself. Therefore, specific procedures for determining a safe and acceptable range for your elevated heart rate are outlined in the walking program at the back of the book. For now, listen to your body. Lengthen your stride slightly when you walk and let your natural body rhythm dictate your walking speed. And remember, the basic elements of walking still apply: GRADUALISM, CONSISTENCY, and ENJOYMENT.

The Fun of It

Walking Up Hills

Hills were made to be enjoyed and conquered, not avoided. Accept them as one of the many challenges facing a serious walker. With this I-can-conquer attitude, you will be able to walk up hills in a matter of weeks without getting out of breath.

It all begins when you include one hill in your daily walk. Decrease your pace several hundred feet away from the hill (or stop completely if you like), breathe deeply several times, and then proceed to attack the hill, slowly and methodically.

Once you are comfortable walking up your first hill, identify several others (slightly steeper of course) along your walking route that you would like to conquer and then set a realistic timetable. To derive additional pleasure from hill climbing, find that special hill . . . one that appeals to you personally. The attraction might be the slope, the way the trees are arched, the view from the top, or just the bouncy exhilarating feeling you get as you descend from it. When you find it you will know.

Now some of you are going to think I'm crazy, but I want you to give that hill a name. Call it Love Hill, Heart Hill, Mini-Mt. Everest, or Energy Incline. Your hill did not start out being special just because it was there. You made it special because you attached some private personal meaning to it. In that sense, the hill belongs to you—so why not give it a name?

Many walkers report that the reason they avoid hills is because they are afraid of overexerting themselves. This fear can be put aside by your setting a slow to moderate pace and then listening to your body. If you are able to carry on a normal conversation with your walking partner—or to recite your favorite poem—then your pace is probably right on target. If, on the other hand, you need to stop and catch your breath, that is a signal to slow down.

Stair Walking

On those days when the weather is inclement and you have chosen one of your indoor sites in order to stay on your regular walking schedule, walk up several flights of stairs toward the end of your walk. Stair walking is a good substitute for your outdoor walk in other special situations as well, such as when you are on vacation and do not want to venture too far from your hotel, or when you attend a convention and forget to bring your walking attire.

Remember that walk I mentioned earlier that I took in a hotel in Atlanta? Something I didn't tell you is that continuous stair walking burns twice as many calories as walking on non-graded surfaces, so I was able to walk off most of the extra calories I had consumed during the convention I was attending. More important, walking the stairs was a refreshing respite from sitting in meetings all day.

Arm Swinging

One way to readily identify serious walkers is to watch them swing their arms. Europeans even assert that you have not walked fast enough until your arms are more tired than your legs. Furthermore, some medical authorities attribute the vigorous use of the upper body to the longer than average life span of symphony conductors. As they rehearse the orchestra and conduct, the use of their arms elevates their heart rate and they receive a cardiovascular workout. If you doubt the authenticity of this statement, stand in place right now and wave your arms back and forth for 2 or 3 minutes. Didn't your heart rate become elevated?

The message, whether you are walking indoors or outdoors, just for FUN or for the HEALTH of it, is: Walk briskly, accept hills as a challenge, include stair climbing when you are walking indoors, and swing those arms!

TIPS FOR INCREASING DAILY WALKING

Perhaps planning when and where you are going to walk and incorporating additional walking into your daily routine will expand the number of benefits you are receiving. I will leave the review of your own walking benefits up to you and simply list below a few tips on ways to increase your walking during the day.

- Do not spend extra time and gas looking for a close parking space at the shopping mall. Park your car as far away as possible in the parking lot and walk to the store.
- Park as far away as possible from your job and walk to your office building. On leaving work, take the longest route possible to get to your car.

- Walk to the neighborhood store instead of sending the children.
- Take a walking break instead of a coffee break. While your co-workers are drinking coffee and having donuts, go for a 10- or 15-minute walk. You will return more refreshed and will save calories and money to boot.
- Take the stairs instead of the escalator or elevator at work or when shopping. If you work or live in a high-rise building, get off the elevator two or three floors before your stop and walk up several flights of stairs.
- Walk to the bus stop to pick up your children after school and walk home with them.
- If you are a member of a car pool responsible for picking up children after school, arrive 5 to 10 minutes early, park the car, and go for a walk instead of sitting in the car waiting for the dismissal of school.
- Become the office walker and memo deliverer and never pass up an opportunity to take something down the hall or to the next floor.
- Go window shopping without your purse.
- When grocery shopping, walk down each aisle and do some comparative shopping first, then return to the entrance of the store and start your shopping.
- Don't use the laundry chute and don't wait until the hamper is full before you empty it. Empty the hamper every day and try to make several trips to the basement each day.
- Take the garbage out after each meal.
- Don't take all of the mail out of the mailbox at one time. Take out one piece, then, an hour later, take out another piece, and so forth.
- Have your husband/wife or the driver in the car pool drop you off and pick you up 3 or 4 blocks from where you work and from your home.
- If you ride the bus, walk to the next stop instead of standing and waiting for the bus.
- Get off the bus several blocks from your destination.

- Walk down to the corner and back while your car is warming up during winter months.
- Answer the telephone in the area of the house farthest from you.
- Walk to work and save money on gas and bus fares.
- If you live in the suburbs and ride the train to the city, walk from your house to the train station.
- On your return from the city, walk on the train platform to the next stop before boarding it for home.

9

Prevention of Injuries and Physical Discomfort

Among the many reasons and excuses formerly enthusiastic walkers give for discontinuing walking are injuries, physical discomfort, boredom, unsafe streets, neighborhood dogs, lack of willpower, bad weather, and no one to walk with. I have already discussed most of these problems and offered tips on ways to handle them, but now we need to focus on one of the most important factors in long-term success: the prevention of injuries and physical discomfort.

Since many of the injuries that occur as a result of walking can be attributed to neglect of body signals (e.g., walking too far or too fast too soon, poor walking style, improper shoes), they can be prevented. In addition, you can assess the degree of discomfort during or after your walk and probably solve any problems yourself. For instance, the next time you think you have hurt yourself or you notice a slight discomfort—either while walking or several hours or days later—don't panic. Become self-reliant. Retrace your steps and systematically analyze the signals that you are receiving from your body. Here are a few questions I might ask you if I were there:

1. Is it pain, discomfort, or soreness?
2. Is it from walking or could it be from some other activity?

3. What is the extent of the discomfort or pain?
4. Is the discomfort or pain localized? Radiating upward or downward?
5. Is it an aggravated old injury?
6. Is this the first time you have had this problem?
7. Did you walk faster or farther yesterday or today?
8. What kind of surface did you walk on?
9. What kind of shoes were you wearing?
10. Did you do any warm-up and cool-down exercises?
11. Have you incorporated stretching exercises into your daily routine?
12. Did you reconsider the basic elements of walking?

A word of caution, though. While all of these factors form the basis for the self-help measures that I am about to recommend, you know your body best. Therefore, if the discomfort persists after retracing your steps, identifying the problem(s) and probable cause(s), and trying the recommendations listed below, see your physician for corrective action and follow his recommendations.

Problem	Probable Cause	Treatment and/or Solution
Heart palpitation	Walking too fast; overexertion; too steep an incline.	Decrease speed; intermittent walking. If palpitation persists, see physician.
Lightheadedness, dizziness	Inadequate circulation to the brain; walking too fast.	Slow down and stop; sit down and lower your head. Contact physician.
Inability to find pulse; fading pulse	Excess fatty tissue at the pulse site; on medication; blood vessels submerged.	Practice finding the most prominent pulse site. Check with physician to see if fading pulse is normal for you.

Problem	Probable Cause	Treatment and/or Solution
Low pulse rate	Good physical condition; on medication; one of small percentage of the population with a low pulse rate.	Check with physician to see what the elevation of your pulse should be while walking.
Breathing difficulty	Shallow breathing; excessive speed, taxing heart and lungs too much; poor posture.	Decrease speed; assess posture and breathing; monitor heart rate more closely; practice deep breathing.
Nausea, pain in rib cage	Walking too fast; exceeding maximum heart rate; lactic acid buildup in the blood.	Slow down and walk at a more modest pace.
Numbness in fingers	Hands and arms not moving and in a dependent position while walking, thus blood pooling in the fingers.	Contract and relax muscles in the hand and arm; tighten fist and release; move hands while walking; elevate hands over head.
Sleeping difficulty	Excessive brisk walking at night; biological clock adjusting to increased activity; less sleep needed.	Break up walking into morning and afternoon sessions; slow relaxing walks at night; warm bath and relaxation exercises before going to bed.
Lower back pain	Walking style; obesity; excess fatty tissue in the abdominal area, pulling upper body back to prevent loss of balance.	Back exercises; increase in warm-up and cool-down exercises and flexibility-stretching exercises; intermittent walking schedule; weight loss.

Problem	Probable Cause	Treatment and/or Solution
Hip pain	Poor body alignment; improper walking style; walking too fast; osteoporosis; early arthritis.	Decrease speed; assess posture and walking style; add hip rotations to warm-up and cool-down routine.
Calf and thigh muscle soreness	Muscle atrophy and disuse; body not accustomed to sustained walking; hard walking surface.	Soak in hot water; gentle massage of lower extremities; extend warm-up and cool-down exercises; decrease walking speed and distance if pain persists.
Thigh chafing	Excess fatty tissue in thigh region; structure of lower extremities; poor walking style; all of the above.	Apply lotion or Vaseline to the inner thighs before walking; wear long pants or shorts that are long enough to prevent thighs from rubbing against each other.
Knee pain	Pushing off too hard on the toes; high toe-off to increase speed; overcompensating with the nondominant leg; early arthritis.	Decrease speed; deemphasize pushing off on toes; concentrate on heel strike; perform knee exercises inside and outside bathtub.
Shin splint	Hard walking surface; poor walking style; low arches; improper shoes.	Walk on grass and asphalt; lower leg exercises, soft arch supports; check shoes.
Ankle injuries	Poor heel strike; improper shoes; worn-over heels; poor body alignment; congenital defects.	Check walking style, surfaces, and shoes.

Problem	Probable Cause	Treatment and/or Solution
Achilles tendon pain	Warm up and cool down too short; traumatization of taut achilles tendon; low heel; high heel; poor heel strike.	Walk slower; perfect walking style and heel strike; check walking surfaces; check shoes; slow down.
Heel spur	Improper shoes; hard rocky walking surfaces; heavy heel strike.	Sponge rubber cushion; corrective shoes with adequate heel cushion; shoes with higher heel elevation; walk on softer surface. See podiatrist if problem persists.
Pain in the heel	Excessive trauma to the heel; low heels; poor walking style and heel impact; hard walking surface; improper shoes.	Check walking style; use outer and inner heel cushion of sponge rubber; use sole and heel pads.
Pain in the instep	Poor arch support; hard walking surface; improper walking style; improper shoes.	Check shoes for proper arch support; check walking surface; check walking style; foot massage and exercises.
Pain in ball of foot	Ill-fitting shoes; improper lining; hard walking surface; worn soles; high toe-off.	Check walking style, especially toe-off; walk on grass or asphalt; intermittent walking, foot massage, and exercises.
Soft corns	Found in the web of opposing toes that exert pressure on each other while walking.	Separate toes with a small sponge-like plaster. See podiatrist if problem persists.

Problem	Probable Cause	Treatment and/or Solution
Hard corns	Ill-fitting shoes; aggravation of old corn.	Corn plaster; roomier shoes. See podiatrist if problem persists.
Bunions	Congenital defect where big toe angulates toward the second toe.	Corrective shoes are recommended with adequate width, flatter heel, and special pouch cut out at the site of the bunion; check arch supports; foot exercises.
Calluses	Ill-fitting shoes; poor walking style; abnormal pressure and friction; enlarged toe joints.	Examine foot; wear roomier shoes; check walking style and walking surfaces.
Blisters	Improper shoes; ill-fitting socks.	Check shoes and socks.
Sore gluteal (buttock) muscles	Walking too fast or too long; overexertion; climbing hills.	Hot soaks; gentle massage; slower walking pace for 2 or 3 days; discontinue walking for a day.

10

Keeping It Going

By reading this book and experiencing what walking is, you have made significant progress toward your initial goal: a more enjoyable, fit, and healthy life. The second goal, now that you are aware of some ways to minimize injuries, is to maximize your probability of success. Simply put, you must utilize all of the strategies mentioned that have worked for you, develop additional strategies of your own, and keep walking until you are permanently and positively addicted. Thus the following information, gleaned from some of the self-reports of successful walkers presented earlier, will be extremely beneficial when you find your interest or motivation for walking subsiding.

Commitment

Commitment is another way of saying *I will,* and is not based on what you should or might do. This "I will" attitude is reflected in the following four-point walking creed:

1. I will schedule my daily activities around my walking and not my walking around my activities.
2. I will make time for walking rather than try to find time for walking.
3. I will go for a walk every day.
4. I will not stand or ride when I can walk.

By repeating this creed to yourself every day, your commitment to walking will remain high.

Not the End, but the Beginning

The mind-set that a walking program is over after 8 to 12 weeks is a frequent trap that many walkers fall into. While it is true that, once you reach your ideal fitness level, you can maintain that level by going for a 45-minute or 1-hour brisk walk three or four times a week, most walkers are not able to make an enduring change in their life-style that quickly. Therefore, after completing the various levels of the program and achieving significant physical, psychological, and financial benefits, your program is not over—a new way of life is just beginning.

Setting a Walking Goal

Another way to keep your walking program going is by setting a short-range (daily, weekly) and/or long-range (monthly, quarterly, semi-annual, annual) walking goal. There are two points worth remembering in this regard. First, your walking goal should be specific. To say, "I will walk down the block several days a week" is too general. A more specific walking goal would be for you to say, "I will go for a 10-minute or a half-mile walk on Monday, Wednesday, and Friday evening."

Second, your walking goal should be realistic. Using the above illustration, you must ask yourself, "Is there a conflict on the days that I indicated I would walk? Will I overdo it if I walk that distance 3 days a week?" If your answer is yes to these questions, your goal is probably unattainable, and thus unrealistic. You are encouraged to set your walking goal high, but to make certain that it is within your reach.

Alternate Plans

While you may not be able to predict the future and develop contingency plans for all circumstances, you can have an alternate plan in the event of inclement weather or if your walking partner does not show up to walk with you. Now is the time to plan ahead and begin thinking about additional places where you can walk when situations arise that are out of your control. Making the adjustment to emergencies is simply a matter of being prepared.

Personal Diary

A diary of your walking experiences can be very inspiring, especially if you like walking alone in rural areas or exploring different areas of your community. What you write is up to you. The naturalist Edwin Teale described the change of season and his observations of animals in their natural habitat in his diary. In addition to writing about nature, you might want to record some of the amusing and unusual events that occur along your walking route, or interesting personalities you met while walking, or your personal feelings and moods, or how you solved a personal problem. Whatever the focus of your diary, forcing yourself to write is not the answer . . . just let the words flow naturally.

Collecting Memorabilia and Reading about Walkers

An excellent hobby that can be reinforcing and motivating is to collect memorabilia of all the different places you have walked. You can also take pictures for a walking scrapbook or make a movie of the various places you have discovered while walking, then show them proudly to your friends and family at social gatherings.

Another way to increase your awareness about the beauty

of walking is to read about famous walkers. As mentioned earlier, some of the most influential figures in the history of the United States were walkers who wrote eloquently on the personal satisfaction derived from walking. In addition, the *Guinness Book of Records* has a section on walking that is very inspiring. But a word of caution: Collecting memorabilia and reading about walking is all for nought if you are not engaged as a walker yourself.

Helping Others

"When I help someone else, I am helping myself." How true! By encouraging others to walk, you will walk more yourself. I learned this for myself when I first started walking to work and began encouraging people waiting for the bus to walk with me for a block or so. After a while I saw more and more people along my route walking instead of waiting for the bus. One of my eventual converts to "bus stop walking" informed me that she was not going to walk between stops because she had tried it several times at my suggestion and had missed her bus more than once. I asked if she had considered walking toward the approaching bus rather than away from it—and now I see her walking 3 or 4 blocks toward the bus many mornings. We always smile and wave at each other as we pass.

If you want to be more formal about encouraging and helping others to walk, you can establish a walking club at your church or in your neighborhood and set aside times when everyone can get together to take a walk. You will profit as much if not more than anyone else since you will be assuming a leadership role in which you take the initiative to plan and develop walking routes and tours for the group. Mobilize the family and make walking a family affair as well. Richard did it.

Richard was 200 pounds overweight at age 30 when he entered my clinical program for weight management. Our group meetings were held on the second floor and he had to stop and rest after climbing each flight of stairs. He began participating in yoga exercises and committed himself to a walking program. He gradually increased his walking over a 1-month period from a quarter of a mile to a mile every morning. Then during the next 3 months he increased his morning walk to 3 miles, still at a slow pace, concentrating on building his endurance and stamina. Richard lost 50 pounds in 6 months. More important, his weight loss and consistent walking lowered his heart rate, decreased his blood pressure, and made him feel less self-conscious about his obese body. He even reported that the more he walked the more clearly he was able to think. He became so addicted to walking that he mobilized his whole family—including an 80-year-old grandmother—for regular neighborhood walks.

The enthusiasm you can generate for walking by helping others is unlimited. Try it. You will soon see that by helping others you will be helping yourself.

Visible Reminders

Any item that you can place in public view to prompt your attention to walking, or that will remind you of your specific commitment or goal, will help maintain your motivation. For instance, I have a corner in my living room near the door that I call my walking corner. This is where I keep my walking sticks, walking hats, raincoat, and other gear for bad weather. Another technique is to lay out your walking-related items each night (shoes, pants, dress, jacket, pedometer, or whatever). In the morning, you do not have to spend time scurrying about the house deciding what you are going to wear. You simply get up, get dressed, do your warm-up exercises, and go for a walk.

Cue cards are also helpful reminders. Write a note to yourself and leave it in a very conspicuous place, e.g., bathroom mirror, dining room table, or refrigerator door. The note might contain an inspirational message about walking

—or it might be more specific, simply reminding you about the special place you plan to walk that day.

Variety

Many people walk the same route day after day, year after year, and never get bored. They seem comfortable with their established route and enjoy walking in this consistent and predictable pattern. If you are one of those people, fine. If, on the other hand, you are prone to boredom, you will have to vary your walking route as well as your schedule in order to keep up your motivation.

Variety can be spontaneous, whereby you deviate one or two blocks from your established route to see another area of your community, or it can be planned. As you drive around the city where you live, or when you visit another city, survey the area to find a good safe place for continuous walking. Write down the location and make it a point to return for a walk.

Try a walking game such as "orienteering" once a month to add variety to your walking program. Orienteering, a game in which you use a compass and a map to locate a hidden treasure in a park or the woods, will increase your overall walking total for the day and is a sport in which your family and friends can participate.

Find a Walking Buddy

The support you receive from your family and friends is important to the ultimate success of your walking program. While verbal encouragement is wonderful, many people find it helpful to walk with another person as well. Make a date to walk with a friend and set up a mutually supportive buddy system. Knowing that someone is counting on you to walk many times is sufficient to force you to live up to your personal commitment even though you might want to cancel the walking date.

Two participants in one of my weight management groups collectively walked 800 miles in 5 months and lost 40 and 50 pounds, respectively. These dedicated walkers walked during the snowy winter of 1978 in Nashville. They walked every day (sometimes after midnight), in the rain and snow, for approximately an hour at a brisk pace. Both women admitted at the end of the program that they would not have walked that distance, or indeed that consistently, without the other. Thus in selecting a walking buddy, make sure that the person needs your support as much as you need his or hers.

Special Events

Participating in special events can be one of your long-range goals. Select a special event several months away and put yourself on a progressive walking schedule. Several events come to mind. One is the Bonne Bell Race for women held every year in many cities throughout the United States. Although the 10-kilometer run (6.2 miles) is advertised for joggers, walkers are participating each year in growing numbers. You can walk at your own speed and receive the physical benefits as well as the T-shirts and cosmetic products that go to all participants who enter the race. A second special event is the Presidential Sports Award that is given for fitness walking. The goal is to walk 125 miles in 50 days. Once you reach a level where you are consistently walking 3 miles a day, send off for the forms, complete the requirements, and you will qualify for a patch, medal, and certificate. (The address is Presidential Sports Award, P.O. Box 706, Old Chelsea Station, New York, NY 10011.)

Cultivate an Appreciation for Silence and Being Alone

From the time you get up in the morning until you drift off to sleep 16 hours later, it is likely that you will be bombarded with noise. Some of the noise pollution in your environment cannot be avoided, but many times you turn on the radio or television to buffer loneliness or to avoid getting in touch with your true feelings. Successful walkers use silence and being alone to enter their private world and meditate, solve a problem, or just let their minds wander freely. In addition, they are able to continue walking alone when their buddy support system breaks down because they have been able to cultivate an appreciation for silence and being alone. Silence is golden only if you appreciate it. And that sometimes takes practice.

THE WALKING PROGRAM

Steps to Developing a Fitness Walking Program

The three major steps involved in developing a fitness walking program are assessment, assignment to an individualized program, and measurement of your progress. Two important procedures related to the above steps are taking your pulse and determining your target heart rate zone.

Taking Your Pulse

Since your heartbeat is about the same as your pulse beat, a simple and convenient way to determine your heart rate at rest and when you are walking is by taking your pulse. There are a number of sites on your body where you can take your pulse. Three of the most common sites are the carotid artery, located along the trachea of your neck about an inch below the jawbone; the radial artery, which is along the inner wrist above the thumb joint; and the temporal artery, found in the temple area. I use the radial artery to take my pulse because this is the site where my pulse is most prominent. This may not be the case with you, however, so you will need to experiment with finding your pulse.

Using your index and middle finger, take a few minutes to feel your pulse at each of the three sites mentioned. You may have to move your finger around slightly in each of these areas before you feel the rhythmic pulsating beat. Once you determine the site at which your pulse beats most strongly, you will need a watch or clock with a sweeping second hand to determine your resting pulse rate or heart rate. With your index finger and middle finger (never your thumb), press down lightly at the identified site. When you feel a rhythmic pulsating beat against your finger, count the number of beats for 15 seconds and then multiply the number by 4. (This is the same as counting each beat for 60 seconds.)

What was your resting heart rate?

Jot the number down and repeat the procedure several times. Were you able to obtain a consistent resting heart rate each time? Since taking your pulse before, during, and after walking is a standard procedure associated with the fitness walking program, continue taking your pulse several times a day.

There are several reasons why taking your pulse for 15 seconds and multiplying by 4 is recommended instead of taking your pulse for a full 60 seconds. For one, your heart rate tends to drop rapidly when you discontinue walking, so in the first 15 seconds you are able to obtain a pulse level that most accurately reflects what your activity level was while you were walking. In addition, the abbreviated procedure gives you immediate feedback on your level of exertion and can be used as a gauge to increase or decrease your walking speed.

Determining Your Target Zone

If you were to run until you were exhausted and then take your pulse, your heart would be beating at its maximal level, perhaps as high as 220 beats per minute. You do not need to elevate your heart rate to its maximal capacity or sustain it at that level in order to receive cardiovascular benefits. What is necessary, though, is to elevate and sustain your heart rate at a level—or in a zone—that is safe and yet will condition your cardiovascular system. A level or zone that is considered safe is 70% to 90% of your maximal heart rate. This is known as your target heart rate zone, or your training level. There are also a number of other terms that are used interchangeably for target heart rate zone, namely, target range and conditioning level. You may also hear such terms as cardiovascular overload, aerobic effects, stimulus period, or cardiovascular workout. Do not let these terms confuse you since they all mean about the same thing.

To determine your target heart rate zone, you must first determine your maximal heart rate. Resting heart rate and maximal heart rate decrease as we get older, so the first step in determining your maximal heart rate is to subtract your age from 220 (the highest attainable heart rate for most people). I will determine my maximal heart rate and would like for you to work along with me to determine yours:

$$
\begin{array}{c}
\quad 220 \text{ (max. heart rate)} \\
\underline{-\quad 42 \text{ (my age)}} \\
\quad 178 \text{ (my max. heart rate)}
\end{array}
\qquad
\begin{array}{c}
\quad 220 \text{ (max. heart rate)} \\
\underline{-\quad\quad \text{ (your age)}} \\
\quad\quad \text{ (your max. heart rate)}
\end{array}
$$

Now that you have determined your maximal heart rate, the next step is to find out your target heart rate zone, which is at 70% and 90% of your maximal capacity. I will compute mine first:

$$
\begin{array}{c}
\quad 178 \\
\underline{\times \quad .70 \text{ (70\%)}} \\
124.60 \text{ (125)}
\end{array}
\qquad
\begin{array}{c}
\quad 178 \\
\underline{\times \quad .90 \text{ (90\%)}} \\
160.20 \text{ (160)}
\end{array}
$$

Thus my target heart rate zone is 125 to 160. Now compute yours in the same way:

$$
\begin{array}{c}
\underline{\quad\quad} \text{ (your max.} \\
\text{heart rate)} \\
\underline{\times .70 \text{ (70\%)}} \\
(\quad)
\end{array}
\qquad
\begin{array}{c}
\underline{\quad\quad} \text{ (your max.} \\
\text{heart rate)} \\
\underline{\times .90 \text{ (90\%)}} \\
(\quad)
\end{array}
$$

Your target heart rate zone is ＿＿＿ to ＿＿＿.

Now that you know how to take your pulse and have

determined your target heart rate zone, please complete the
following statements for easy reference later:

My most prominent pulse site is my _____ artery.
My resting heart rate (pulse) is _____.
My maximal heart rate (corrected for my age) is _____.
My target heart rate zone is _____ to _____.

There are many factors (e.g., sex, medication, climate,
mental state, time of day, and level of fitness) that may
influence your heart rate at rest and your maximal heart rate.
However, in most cases, elevating your heart rate to 70% to
90% of its maximal capacity and sustaining it at that level
for a specified period of time is sufficient to condition your
cardiovascular system.

Step 1. Assessment

The purpose of assessment is to answer the following
questions: How fast, how far, and how often should you
walk to receive cardiovascular benefits? How much pain,
if any, do you experience while walking? The following
walking test is designed not only to assess your cardiovascular response to walking at different rates of speed, but
to make sure that you begin with a walking program that
is safe and tolerable. The test consists of walking for 5 minutes at 3 miles per hour, continued walking at 5-minute
intervals at 3½ and 4 miles per hour, and brisk walking at
4½ to 5 miles per hour for an additional 5 minutes. Everyone
is not expected to complete all sections of the test since the
cardiovascular response to walking will differ for each individual.

Attire for the Test

You should wear loose, comfortable clothes that are appropriate for the weather and comfortable shoes that will

permit you to walk for 20 minutes if necessary without discomfort.

Equipment Needed

The only items you will need besides comfortable clothes and shoes are a watch with a second hand, a pencil, and a piece of paper. These items are needed so that you can jot down certain information as you complete the test.

A WORD OF CAUTION

If you experience pain in your joints, muscle cramps or soreness, difficulty in breathing, dizziness, nausea, or any other unusual symptom at any point during the test, STOP, take your pulse, and discontinue the test. Do not go above the midpoint of your target heart rate zone.

Initial Walking Test

Before you begin the walking test, take your pulse and record your resting heart rate. If you are unable to walk for 5 minutes, walk as far as you can at a moderate pace, then stop, take your pulse, and complete the Pain Index and the Post-Walking Assessment, both of which follow the walking tests.

5-Minute Walk at 3 Miles per Hour

Start walking slowly on a level surface and set your pace at about 90 steps a minute, which is a rough approximation of walking at 3 miles per hour. After you have established your pace, walk at that rate of speed for 5 minutes. At 5 minutes, STOP, take your pulse for 15 seconds, and multiply by 4. Jot down your pulse rate. If it is approaching the midpoint of your target heart rate zone, discontinue the test and complete the Pain Index and Post-Walking Assessment.

5-Minute Walk at 3½ Miles per Hour

Continue walking and increase your walking pace to 110 steps a minute, which is approximately 3½ miles an hour. After you have established this pace, walk at that rate for 5 minutes and swing your arms slightly back and forth. At the end of 5 minutes, STOP, take your pulse for 15 seconds, and multiply by 4. Jot down your pulse rate. If it is approaching the midpoint of your target heart rate zone, discontinue the test and complete the Pain Index and Post-Walking Assessment.

5-Minute Walk at 4 Miles per Hour

Continue walking and increase your pace to 125 steps a minute, which is approximately 4 miles per hour. Swing your arms 6 inches forward and 3 inches backward as you walk. At the end of 5 minutes, STOP, take your pulse for 15 seconds, multiply by 4, and jot down your pulse rate. If it is above the midpoint of your target zone, discontinue the test and complete the Pain Index and Post-Walking Assessment.

Additional 5-Minute Walk at 4 Miles per Hour

Continue walking at the 4 mile pace. If you are not able to continue the full 5 minutes, indicate the number of minutes that you walked at this level and complete the Pain Index and Post-Walking Assessment.

At this point, you have been walking for 20 minutes at varying rates of speed. If you have not gotten your heart rate elevated to within your target zone at this point, you are either in good condition or you are taking some form of medication to suppress your heart rate. The next test is for those who are not taking medication and have not experienced any pain the past 20 minutes.

5- to 10-Minute Walk at 4½ to 5 Miles per Hour

Take 3 minutes to build your speed and then walk as fast as you can for up to 10 minutes. STOP, take your pulse, indicate the number of minutes you walked at this pace, and then complete the Pain Index and Post-Walking Assessment.

PAIN INDEX

Area	Left Moderate	Left Severe	Right Moderate	Right Severe
Upper Back				
Lower Back				
Hip				
Thigh				
Knee				
Calf				
Shin				
Ankle				
Instep/Arch				
Achilles Tendon				
Heel				
Ball of Foot				

POST-WALKING ASSESSMENT

Date _____

Age _____ Sex _____ Height _____ Weight _____

Resting Heart Rate (Pulse) _____

Maximal Heart Rate (Pulse) _____

Target Heart Rate Zone _____ to _____

5-minute walk (3 mph)	_____ number of minutes	_____ heart rate (pulse)
5-minute walk (3½ mph)	_____ number of minutes	_____ heart rate (pulse)
5-minute walk (4 mph)	_____ number of minutes	_____ heart rate (pulse)
5-minute walk (4½ mph)	_____ number of minutes	_____ heart rate (pulse)
5 to 10 minute walk (4½ to 5½ mph)	_____ number of minutes	_____ heart rate (pulse)

Before considering your Post-Walking Assessment, take a moment and review your Pain Index. Did you experience pain in any of the areas listed? If so, which area? And what was the degree of discomfort? Was the pain related to an old injury? Mentally retracing your steps and asking questions of this nature are very important. It may well be, depending on the severity of the pain, that you will have to walk at a slower pace initially, or begin with a program at a lower level. It might also be helpful to read or reread Chapter 9 on common injuries and to try some of the recommendations therein.

Now turn to your Post-Walking Assessment. The principal factor that determines your assignment to a specific walking program is your cardiovascular response to walking, that is, how fast and how long you had to walk to elevate your heart rate into your target zone. This is a very important consideration since you want to begin your program at a safe and tolerable level of exertion. Later, as your level of fitness improves, information on your Post-Walking Assessment will assist you in measuring the degree of improvement.

Step 2. Assignment to
Individualized Walking Programs

If you were unable to walk continuously for 5 minutes, you should start with the **Red Program.** If it took 5 minutes of walking at 3 miles per hour for you to reach your target zone, you should begin with the **Blinking Red Program.** For the **Yellow Program,** you should have reached your target zone after walking 5 minutes at 3 miles per hour and 5 minutes at 3½ miles per hour. To enter the **Blinking Green Program** you should have been able to engage in brisk walking at 4 miles per hour for 5 to 10 minutes before reaching your target zone. Finally, the **Green Program** is for those of you who demonstrated that a brisk walking speed of 4 miles per hour for more than 10 minutes was needed to elevate your heart rate into your target zone.

Each 3-week program takes into consideration three factors: intensity, duration, and frequency. As far as intensity is concerned, the results of your walking test are your guide. You should walk at a rate of speed that will elevate your heart rate into your target zone. The length of time (duration) that you should walk will vary across each program. But, irrespective of the program, you should sustain your heart rate in your target zone for a specified period of time. Then, each week, gradually and consistently increase the number of minutes that you keep your heart rate sustained in your target zone. Your long-range goal is to keep your heart rate elevated for 20 to 30 minutes.

With respect to the question of how frequently you should walk, exercise physiologists have determined that walking at least 3 days a week is needed to achieve and maintain fitness benefits. Thus, consistent with the 3-day-a-week minimum requirement, the programs outlined below are based on a hard/easy approach. That is, during a 1-week period, 3 days will be your "hard days," which means that you will set a specific period of time for fitness walking. On alternate days, your "easy days," you will still be expected to go for a walk at a moderate pace and continue incorporating walking into your daily schedule.

A final concern, now that you have been assigned to a walking program, is warm up and cool down. This refers to flexibility exercises prior to and immediately after your fitness walk. Let me illustrate their importance: If the temperature were 10 degrees below zero and you had your car parked overnight, would you start it and drive away without warming it up? Probably not. The human body needs to begin making the adjustment for fitness walking in a similar manner, so you should warm up your body before you begin your walk. By performing, slowly and methodically, the stretching exercises listed below for 5 to 10 minutes prior to walking, you will increase the circulation of your blood, elevate your heart rate slightly, and raise your body temperature. Stretching exercises during this preparatory period also increase the flexibility of your joints and the elasticity of your muscles—both important aids in the prevention of injuries.

Then too, stopping abruptly and sitting down immediately upon completing your fitness walk can result in pooling of blood in the legs and feet, tightening of the muscles, and stiffening of the joints. To prevent these possible aftereffects, begin decreasing your walking speed several blocks before the end of your walk. This will allow your body systems (heart rate and body temperature) to return to their normal state. Once you are inside, continue pacing slowly or perform some household chores standing up for a few minutes (avoiding your easy chair at all cost), then do 5 to 10 minutes of stretching exercises to relax your tense muscles.

For all of the reasons stated above, the following stretching exercises are recommended before and after each fitness walk on your hard days. They should also be incorporated into your easy but active days.

Stretching and Flexibility Exercises

EXERCISE I: Head and Neck Rotation

Turn your head to the right as far as possible and hold that position for 5 seconds; return to forward position and relax.

Turn your head to the left as far as possible and hold that position for 5 seconds; return to forward position and relax.

Rotate your head slowly in a circle, first to the right 5 times, then to the left 5 times.

Relax and breathe deeply several times.

EXERCISE II: Rag Doll

Raise your arms above your head and take a slow, lazy stretch, reaching up as high as possible and going up on your toes. Hold this position until the count of 3, then slowly come down on your heels.

Bend your body over and let it hang. Do not try to touch your toes and do not bounce; just let your body hang lazily, like a rag doll, and count 10.

Repeat this exercise 2 more times, each time slowly, and let your body hang both times for a count of 10.

EXERCISE III: Waist Twist

Place your feet approximately 12 inches apart and swing your arms lazily from side to side, twisting from the waist and looking as far behind you as possible on each side.

Repeat this 10 times; each time should take approximately 6 seconds.

EXERCISE IV: Side Body Bend

Clasp your hands over your head and turn palms upward.

Take a deep breath, bend from your waist to your left as far as possible, exhale, and then straighten up.

Inhale and bend to the right as far as possible, exhale, straighten up.

Inhale and lean back as far as possible, exhale, straighten up.

Repeat this exercise 3 times in each direction.

EXERCISE V: Knee Lift

Raise your right leg off the floor, reach down with both hands and grab your right knee, then pull your knee up toward your chest. Hold for a count of 3.

Do the same thing with your left leg and knee.

Repeat with each leg and knee 5 times.

EXERCISE VI: Thigh Stretch

With your left hand on a chair or some other object to maintain your balance, lift your right leg off the floor and curl your lower leg behind you. Reach behind you and grasp your instep of your right foot with your right hand and hold your lower leg in that position for 10 seconds. (If you are unable to grasp your foot, grab the bottom of your pants leg.)

Repeat this procedure with the left leg.

Grab and hold each leg 2 times.

EXERCISE VII: Lower Body Squat

Hold both arms straight out in front of you and squat as low as possible, keeping your feet flat on the floor; hold to a count of 3. (If you have difficulty doing this exercise, hold onto a chair and squat as low as possible.)

Repeat this exercise 3 times.

Ready, Set, Go!

It is time to begin your 3-week fitness walking program. Find the one that was indicated for you on the basis of the initial walking tests (**Red, Blinking Red, Yellow, Blinking Green,** or **Green**) and follow the instructions given at the top of that particular program description.

On your hard days (your fitness walking days), take your pulse and record it:

- before you begin your warm-up exercises
- before you begin your walk
- midway through your walk (more times if necessary) to see if your heart rate is in your target zone
- immediately after you complete your walk
- 3 minutes after completing your cool-down exercises

RED PROGRAM

Since you were unable to walk continuously for 5 minutes, concentrate on increasing your endurance for the next 3 weeks. On your hard days (Days 1,3,5) do flexibility exercises I,II, and III to warm up your body before your 5- to 10-minute walk, and repeat the same exercises to cool down. On your easy days (Days 2, 4, 6, 7) spend 5 to 10 minutes doing the same flexibility exercises and increase the number of repetitions. Walk at a slow to moderate pace on your hard days and take your pulse at the times specified under READY, SET, GO!

Day	Week 1		Week 2		Week 3	
1	Warm up	2 minutes	Warm up	2 minutes	Warm up	3 minutes
	WALK	5 to 10 minutes	WALK	5 to 10 minutes	WALK	8 to 12 minutes
	Cool down	2 minutes	Cool down	2 minutes	Cool down	3 minutes
2	Flexibility exercises	5 to 10 minutes	Flexibility exercises	5 to 10 minutes	Flexibility exercises	6 to 12 minutes

3	Warm up WALK Cool down	2 minutes 5 to 10 minutes 2 minutes	Warm up WALK Cool down	3 minutes 8 to 12 minutes 3 minutes
4	Flexibility exercises	5 to 10 minutes	Flexibility exercises	6 to 12 minutes
5	Warm up WALK Cool down	2 minutes 5 to 10 minutes 2 minutes	Warm up WALK Cool down	3 minutes 8 to 12 minutes 3 minutes
6	Flexibility exercises	5 to 10 minutes	Flexibility exercises	6 to 12 minutes
7	Flexibility exercises	5 to 10 minutes	SEE SECTION ON MEASURING YOUR PROGRESS	

BLINKING RED PROGRAM

The 3-week Blinking Red program, which is a "Stop and Go" program, is designed to get you to gradually increase your walking distance without elevating your heart rate above your target heart rate zone. Therefore, on your hard days (Days 1, 3, 5) do flexibility exercises I through IV to warm up your body. Then walk slowly the first 3 to 5 minutes, increase your pace for 3 to 5 minutes, and walk slowly again for the final 3 to 5 minutes. If you find this schedule too taxing, walk for a shorter period of time twice a day. On your easy days (Days 2, 4, 6, 7) do flexibility exercises I through V for 8 to 12 minutes. Take your pulse on your hard days at the times specified under READY, SET, GO!

Day	Week 1		Week 2		Week 3	
1	Warm up	3 minutes	Warm up	3 minutes	Warm up	4 minutes
	WALK	10 to 15 minutes	WALK	12 to 18 minutes	WALK	12 to 20 minutes
	Cool down	3 minutes	Cool down	3 minutes	Cool down	4 minutes
2	Flexibility exercises	8 to 12 minutes	Flexibility exercises	8 to 12 minutes	Flexibility exercises	10 to 15 minutes

3	Warm up 3 minutes WALK 10 to 15 minutes Cool down 3 minutes	Warm up 3 minutes WALK 12 to 18 minutes Cool down 3 minutes	Warm up 4 minutes WALK 12 to 20 minutes Cool down 4 minutes
4	Flexibility exercises 8 to 12 minutes	Flexibility exercises 8 to 12 minutes	Flexibility exercises 10 to 15 minutes
5	Warm up 3 minutes WALK 10 to 15 minutes Cool down 3 minutes	Warm up 3 minutes WALK 12 to 18 minutes Cool down 3 minutes	Warm up 4 minutes WALK 12 to 20 minutes Cool down 4 minutes
6	Flexibility exercises 8 to 12 minutes	Flexibility exercises 8 to 12 minutes	Flexibility exercises 10 to 15 minutes
7	Flexibility exercises 8 to 12 minutes	Flexibility exercises 8 to 12 minutes	SEE SECTION ON MEASURING YOUR PROGRESS

YELLOW PROGRAM

Even though your walking test results indicate that you can engage in a continuous walking program for 10 to 15 minutes without overexerting yourself, you should proceed with caution. Your goal for the next 3 weeks is not only to increase your walking speed and distance gradually but also to elevate and sustain your heart rate in your target zone for 3 to 8 minutes on your hard days (Days 1, 3, 5). Thus, for the first 5 to 8 minutes, walk at 3 miles per hour, increase your walking pace to 3½ miles per hour for 3 to 8 minutes to reach your target zone, and taper off the last 3 to 8 minutes and reduce your speed to 3 miles an hour. Take your pulse on your hard days at the times specified under READY, SET, GO! and do flexibility exercises I through V for your warm-up and cool-down routine. In addition to doing flexibility exercises on your easy days (Days 2, 4, 6, 7) begin incorporating additional walking during the day after the first week and include at least one fun walk at a leisurely pace on Day 6 or 7. Proceed with caution!

Day	Week 1		Week 2		Week 3	
1	Warm up	4 minutes	Warm up	4 minutes	Warm up	5 minutes
	WALK	15 to 20 minutes	WALK	15 to 25 minutes	WALK	20 to 30 minutes
	Cool down	4 minutes	Cool down	4 minutes	Cool down	5 minutes
2	Flexibility exercises	12 to 18 minutes	Flexibility exercises; additional walking during day		Flexibility exercises; additional walking during day	

3	Warm up 4 minutes WALK 15 to 20 minutes Cool down 4 minutes	Warm up 4 minutes WALK 15 to 25 minutes Cool down 4 minutes	Warm up 5 minutes WALK 20 to 30 minutes Cool down 5 minutes
4	Flexibility exercises 12 to 18 minutes	Flexibility exercises; additional walking during day	Flexibility exercises additional walking during day
5	Warm up 4 minutes WALK 15 to 20 minutes Cool down 4 minutes	Warm up 4 minutes WALK 15 to 25 minutes Cool down 4 minutes	Warm up 5 minutes WALK 20 to 30 minutes Cool down 5 minutes
6	Flexibility exercises 12 to 18 minutes	Flexibility exercises; fun walk	Flexibility exercises 12 to 18 minutes
7	Flexibility exercises 12 to 18 minutes	Flexibility exercises 12 to 18 minutes	SEE SECTION ON MEASURING YOUR PROGRESS

BLINKING GREEN PROGRAM

On your hard days (Days 1, 3, 5) begin walking at 3 to 3½ miles an hour for the first 10 minutes, increase your speed to 4 miles an hour the next 5 to 15 minutes, and then reduce your walking pace to 3 to 3½ miles an hour for the final 5 to 10 minutes. Walking at 4 miles an hour should elevate your heart rate into your target zone, but the main objective for the next 3 weeks is to increase the number of minutes that you sustain your elevated heart rate. Do flexibility exercises I through VI for 2 weeks, increasing the number of repetitions the third week, and take your pulse on your hard days at the times specified under READY, SET, GO! Your easy days (Days 2, 4, 6, 7) after the first week should consist of flexibility exercises, additional walks during the day at a brisk pace, and incorporating stretching exercises into your daily routine. It may be difficult to sustain an elevated heart rate for 5 to 15 minutes if this is your initial 3-week program. Persevere and continue with this program until your body adjusts to this additional overload.

Day	Week 1		Week 2		Week 3	
1	Warm up	5 minutes	Warm up	5 minutes	Warm up	7 minutes
	WALK	20 to 30 minutes	WALK	25 to 35 minutes	WALK	25 to 40 minutes
	Cool down	5 minutes	Cool down	5 minutes	Cool down	7 minutes
2	Flexibility exercises	15 to 25 minutes	Flexibility exercises; additional walking during day		Flexibility exercises; additional walking during day	

3	Warm up — 5 minutes WALK — 20 to 30 minutes Cool down — 5 minutes	Warm up — 5 minutes WALK — 25 to 35 minutes Cool down — 5 minutes	Warm up — 7 minutes WALK — 25 to 40 minutes Cool down — 7 minutes
4	Flexibility exercises — 15 to 25 minutes	Flexibility exercises; stair climbing; walking up hills at moderate pace	Flexibility exercises; stair climbing; walking up hills at moderate pace
5	Warm up — 5 minutes WALK — 20 to 30 minutes Cool down — 5 minutes	Warm up — 5 minutes WALK — 25 to 35 minutes Cool down — 5 minutes	Warm up — 7 minutes WALK — 25 to 40 minutes Cool down — 7 minutes
6	Flexibility exercises; fun walk	Flexibility exercises; additional walking during day	Flexibility exercises; fun walk
7	Flexibility exercises	Flexibility exercises; fun walk	SEE SECTION ON MEASURING YOUR PROGRESS

GREEN PROGRAM

You should begin increasing your warm-up and cool-down period the first week since you will be making additional demands on your body. Therefore, on your hard days (Days 1, 3, 5) do all of the flexibility exercises and increase the number of repetitions after the first week. Begin walking at a moderate to brisk pace for 10 to 15 minutes, sustain your elevated heart rate in your target zone for 10 to 20 minutes, and then reduce your walking pace the final 10 to 15 minutes. Take your pulse on your hard days at the times specified under READY, SET, GO! In addition to daily flexibility exercises on your easy days (Days 2, 4, 6, 7), quicken your pace during the day and incorporate flexibility exercises into your daily routine. If this is your initial 3-week program do not become discouraged if you are unable to sustain an elevated heart rate for 10 to 20 minutes after 3 weeks. Continue increasing your walking speed and/or distance over the next 6 to 9 weeks until you are able to sustain an elevated heart rate for 20 to 30 minutes.

Day	Week 1			Week 2			Week 3		
1	Warm up	8 minutes		Warm up	10 minutes		Warm up	10 minutes	
	WALK	30 to 40 minutes		WALK	35 to 45 minutes		WALK	35 to 50 minutes	
	Cool down	8 minutes		Cool down	10 minutes		Cool down	10 minutes	

	Week 1	Week 2	Week 3
2	Flexibility exercises — 20 to 30 minutes	Flexibility exercises; brisk short walk	Flexibility exercises; brisk short walks
3	Warm up 8 minutes / WALK 30 to 40 minutes / Cool down 8 minutes	Warm up 10 minutes / WALK 35 to 45 minutes / Cool down 10 minutes	Warm up 10 minutes / WALK 35 to 50 minutes / Cool down 10 minutes
4	Flexibility exercises — 20 to 30 minutes	Flexibility exercises; stair climbing	Flexibility exercises; stair climbing
5	Warm up 8 minutes / WALK 30 to 40 minutes / Cool down 8 minutes	Warm up 10 minutes / WALK 35 to 45 minutes / Cool down 10 minutes	Warm up 10 minutes / WALK 35 to 50 minutes / Cool down 10 minutes
6	Flexibility exercises; fun walk	Flexibility exercises; active easy day	Flexibility exercises; active easy day
7	Flexibility exercises; active easy day	Flexibility exercises; fun walk	SEE SECTION ON MEASURING YOUR PROGRESS

Step 3. Measuring Your Progress

Now that you have been following a systematic program for 3 weeks, this is a good time to see if your cardiovascular condition has improved. Since the intensity, duration, and frequency of walking influence your heart rate at rest, you can use the heart rates that you obtained and jotted down before walking on your hard days to measure your progress.

Assuming you have been monitoring your pulse 3 days a week, you should have at least 9 pulse readings for the 3-week period. It is unlikely that you will see a change from each recorded pulse to the next, so you should select one hard day each week that will serve to measure your progress. For example, if you have chosen Monday, Wednesday, and Friday as your hard days, you might select Wednesday as the day you will use to compare your progress from one week to another. Consistency is very important, so take a few minutes now to select your measurement day.

Using the data from your measurement day, you can chart your resting heart rate each week on a graph. The sample graph that appears on the next page is similar to the one you constructed earlier to chart your walking mileage and can be used as a model. The weekly resting heart rate for the walker whose performance is illustrated on the graph decreased over the 3-week period, indicating improvement in this walker's cardiovascular condition. Week 1, the walker's resting pulse was 92; Week 2 it was 88; Week 3 it was 85.

Take time out now to construct your own cardiovascular improvement graph. Plot your resting pulse for Week 1, Week 2, and Week 3, then connect these points with straight lines.

Do you see any cardiovascular improvement? If not, do not despair. On your next walk, monitor your pulse to see if you are obtaining an accurate pulse reading, then persist. Within a week or so, you will see changes in your cardiovascular condition.

CARDIOVASCULAR IMPROVEMENT GRAPH

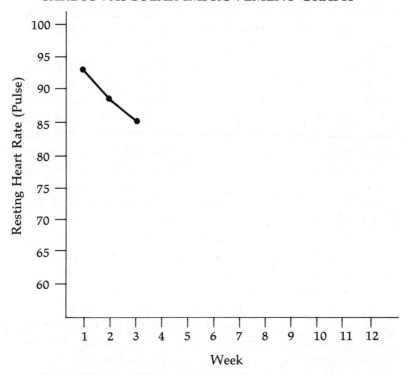

Another indicator that can be used to measure your progress is your performance on the initial walking test. But to use this indicator as a gauge to assess the degree of cardiovascular improvement, you must retake the test. This indicator does not always change immediately, so it is better to retake the initial test after 3 weeks. Even then, the change might be slight, but since you have been walking for 3 weeks, go ahead and retest yourself right now.

First review the information on your Post-Walking Assessment. You will see that you were able to walk X minutes at varying rates of speed. You should now retake the test at the same intensity as before, stopping at the same point at which you had to stop 3 weeks ago. If possible, retake the test on the same day of the week, at the same time of day, walk the same route, and take the specified number of steps for each 5-minute walk. Here, a sign of cardiovascular improvement will be a lower pulse each time you retake the test.

Not everyone will show such a decrease in activity-related heart rate after engaging in a 3-week program of fitness walking, but there are a number of factors that may influence the degree of change. For example, if you are taking medication to suppress your heart rate, brisk walking may elevate your pulse only slightly or not at all. Then, too, there may be some procedural error. Did you retest yourself in exactly the same manner as before? Did you count your pulse for 14 to 16 seconds instead of 15 as recommended? Another factor that may influence how much these indicators change is your initial 3-week program. If you started with the **Red Program**, it may well be that you will see dramatic changes after 3 weeks, whereas those of you who started with the **Yellow Program** might not see any change at all. Thus change in the degree of cardiovascular fitness is relative to your initial cardiovascular response to walking: Persons starting at a lower level of fitness will see greater initial changes than those starting at a higher level of fitness. But you must persist. As you gradually and consistently increase the demands on your body and progress to a higher program level, substantial changes in both your resting heart rate and your cardiovascular response to walking will occur.

Are you ready to move to another program level? Has your body adjusted to your walking intensity, duration, and frequency? If you are able to do more physical work with less effort, or if you are not as tired after you finish walking your predetermined route and would like to walk farther, you are probably ready for another program. You cannot, however, accept these changes at face value. The best way to determine if you are, in fact, ready for a higher level program is to try the first week of that program.

Do not become discouraged if you are unable to walk at

the recommended pace for the period of time specified for the first week of a new program. Since walking at a safe and tolerable level is your main concern, rather than quick progression, repeat the first week until you are comfortable with your progress. Then go to Week 2 and follow the program outlined.

For those of you who started with the **Blinking Green** or **Green Program**, your program does not end after 3 or 6 weeks just because a structured program is not outlined for you. This simply means that your initial level of fitness was higher, therefore you have more latitude in developing an individualized program. The major criterion for cardiovascular fitness, however, remains the same—sustaining your elevated heart rate for 20 to 30 minutes in your target zone. This may not be as easy as it sounds since your body has also adjusted to your present level of fitness. So, when you complete the **Green Program,** experiment with a new and higher level of overload and continue to make additional demands on your body until your pulse (resting and walking heart rate) begins to gradually level off. Only then are you ready to consider new ways to maintain your cardiovascular fitness gains.

IMPORTANT POINTS TO REMEMBER

- Take your resting heart rate bofore going for a walk on your hard days, then continue monitoring your pulse during your walk to make sure it is in your target zone.
- Select one of your hard days as your measurement day and use your resting heart rate from that day to monitor your weekly progress by plotting the information on your graph.
- Review your weekly progress graph to assess the degree of cardiovascular improvement after 3 weeks before committing yourself to a more demanding program. If

your pulse has been decreasing in a consistent manner and you are comfortable with your progress, try the first week of the next program.

Step 4. Maintaining Your Walking Fitness Gains

There are three questions related to your fitness gains that are of interest at this point: How do you maintain your fitness gains? How do you get back on track when your walking schedule is interrupted? How do you attain a higher level of fitness? Let me answer these questions as succinctly as possible.

Your walking fitness gains are reversible, which means that your walking fitness level will deteriorate over time unless you continue walking. For those of you who are approaching or have reached a peak fitness level, the minimal requirement for maintenance is straightforward: You must continue to sustain your elevated heart rate in your target zone for 20 to 30 minutes at least 3 times a week. There may be others of you who have not reached your peak condition but who are walking for a shorter period of time at a comfortable pace and who are not interested in making additional demands on your body—at least at the present time. All that is required is for you to continue walking at your present level and monitor your pulse rate periodically. Being satisfied with your fitness walking accomplishments is just as important as achieving peak physical fitness.

To get back on track, you must consider the effects that discontinuing walking will have on you, physically and mentally. And since your fitness gains are reversible, the longer you discontinue walking, the longer it will take to regain the conditioning effects . . . but it can be done. One way, depending on the number of days or weeks that your walking program has been interrupted, is to go for a leisurely stroll, listen to your body, and gauge the increase in your walking pace and distance accordingly. Another way to get back on track is to retake the initial walking test, assign yourself to the proper program, and assess your improvement after 3 weeks. Whatever the case, do not attempt to regain your former level of fitness too quickly. As a general rule of thumb, it takes twice as long to recover fully after your schedule has been interrupted as the amount of time that has elapsed since that interruption.

While you can revert to a lower level to get back on track physically, the mental perspective is not as straightforward . . . but it can be done! Walking had a high priority before and it can be a high priority in your life again. The best recommendation is to encourage you to reread this book. Perhaps reading about successful walkers, walking aids, or walking benefits will motivate you to recapture some of your walking experience. You may also find the chapter on keeping it going helpful. But more than anything else, a simple resolve is needed. Just say *I can.* Bouncing back and getting on track after a slight setback is the true test of a lifelong committed walker.

It is not surprising that some of you are interested in attaining a higher level of fitness. This is one of the amazing qualities of the human mind and body. The more you do, the more you find that you can do and want to do.

There are several options that you might consider at this point. You may wish to continue focusing on cardiovascular fitness and being a walk-jog program or engage in some other forms of continuous activity to sustain your elevated heart rate. Another option is the total fitness approach in which you might begin an activity program that includes specific exercises to increase your flexibility, muscular strength, body coordination, and cardiovascular condition. A third option is to take it one step at a time and maintain your walking program at its present level. This would be your core physical activity program. And since you have been doing flexibility exercises as part of your warm-up and cool-down routine, you might want to enroll in a formal yoga class to increase your flexibility. Once you have made substantial progress in this area, move on to something else, keeping walking as your mainstay. Always remember, irrespective of the option that you choose to attain a higher level of fitness, that the gradual and consistent approach is best.